D1544763

Prescriptions for the Mind

Prescriptions for the Mind

A Critical View of Contemporary Psychiatry

JOEL PARIS, MD

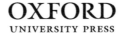

OXFORD

UNIVERSITY PRESS

2008

BP 53

OXFORD
UNIVERSITY PRESS

Oxford University Press, Inc., publishes works that further
Oxford University's objective of excellence
in research, scholarship, and education.

Oxford   New York
Auckland   Cape Town   Dar es Salaam   Hong Kong   Karachi
Kuala Lumpur   Madrid   Melbourne   Mexico City   Nairobi
New Delhi   Shanghai   Taipei   Toronto

With offices in
Argentina   Austria   Brazil   Chile   Czech Republic   France   Greece
Guatemala   Hungary   Italy   Japan   Poland   Portugal   Singapore
South Korea   Switzerland   Thailand   Turkey   Ukraine   Vietnam

Published by Oxford University Press, Inc.
198 Madison Avenue, New York, New York 10016

www.oup.com

Oxford is a registered trademark of Oxford University Press

Library of Congress Cataloging-in-Publication Data
Paris, Joel, 1940–
Prescriptions for the mind : a critical view of contemporary psychiatry / Joel Paris.
p. ; cm.
Includes bibliographical references and index.
ISBN 978-0-19-531383-3
1. Psychiatry—Philosophy.   2. Psychotherapy—Methodology.
[DNLM: 1. Psychiatry—methods.   2. Mental Disorders.   WM 100 P231p 2008]   I. Title.
RC437.5.P37 2008
616.89001—dc22   2008006681

3 5 7 9 8 6 4 2

Printed in the United States of America
on acid-free paper

7/22/10

This book is dedicated to Leon Eisenberg.

Contents

Acknowledgments

I would like to thank Roz Paris and Ned Shorter, who read earlier versions of this book and made many useful suggestions for improvement, and also Leon Eisenberg, Maurice Dongier, Richard U'ren, and Hallie Zweig-Frank, who offered helpful comments on early drafts of several chapters.

A special thanks to my editor at Oxford, Marion Osmun, who believed in this book and took the time to work with me on its shape and contents.

Introduction

Two Visions of Psychiatry

Psychiatrists are experts on the mind and its maladies. But no one is quite sure anymore what it is they do.

It is not surprising that the public has difficulty understanding the field. Psychiatrists themselves are confused about how they should practice.

The discipline remains divided between two visions, and there is a continuing struggle within psychiatry about its future role. Should psychiatrists be more like neurologists—examining patients, making diagnoses, and prescribing drugs? Or should they be more like psychologists—probing the inner workings of the mind and providing expert psychotherapy?

These contrasting visions are not new. In a book published fifty years ago, a sociologist, August Hollingshead, and a psychiatrist, Fritz Redlich, described two types of psychiatrists (Hollingshead and Redlich, 1958). One wore white coats and treated patients in hospitals; the other wore sports jackets and treated patients with psychotherapy in offices. Twenty years later, when I studied psychiatry, my teachers could easily be separated into these two camps.

A seminal article in the *British Journal of Psychiatry* in 1986 by the Harvard psychiatrist Leon Eisenberg, entitled "Mindlessness and Brainlessness in Psychiatry," followed by other publications, critically examined both approaches (Eisenberg, 1986, 1995, 2000). Eisenberg labeled the psychiatry of the past—one that relied on the speculative theory of psychoanalysis—"brainless" because it did not give any serious attention to neuroscience. He was equally critical of a psychiatry that simply saw mental illness as disorders of the brain; a view he labeled "mindless."[1]

In short, both visions are too narrow. Mental illness cannot be understood without taking both biology and psychology into account. In that way, psychiatrists are unique. They are almost the only practitioners who regularly treat patients with combinations of biological and psychological interventions.

Unfortunately, the complexity of the real world runs counter to the preference of the human mind for simplicity. Most people find it easier to think that diseases have single causes. Yet direct and linear relationships between risk factors and actual illness are very rare. One of the themes of this book is that to carry out its mission, psychiatry must embrace complexity.

The Public Image of Psychiatry

Every month, scientific findings in the field of psychiatry appear in top journals and are summarized and discussed in leading newspapers and magazines. Many educated people are familiar with the latest research in the field. In recent years, the media have highlighted biological findings in psychiatry, and one gets the impression that the neurosciences are about to solve the mystery of mental illness. Psychiatrists also seem to believe this. They have become much more biological in their thinking and their practice, and their encounters with patients have come to focus more and more on drug prescriptions.

As psychiatry has changed, so has its public image. Even today, some people see psychiatrists as psychotherapists and are unsure how they differ from psychologists. To counter this confusion, psychiatry has defined itself firmly as a medical specialty. As we will see, this choice of identity has had vast implications.

The Couch and the Prescription Pad

For many years the most familiar symbol of psychiatry was the analytic couch. Readers of *New Yorker* cartoons can attest that the stereotype remains alive and well. But few psychiatrists today are psychoanalysts, and only some psychoanalysts are psychiatrists. Those who practice talk therapies see patients in an armchair, face-to-face. Many psychiatrists, however, never practice formal psychotherapy. Like other physicians, their primary tool is a prescription pad.

As the biological model of mental illness triumphed, talk therapies were marginalized. In a previous book, I examined the decline of psychoanalysis and its dramatic fall from grace within academic psychiatry (Paris, 2005a). With psychoanalysis a fallen icon, what role was left for talk therapies? Unfortunately, a healthy baby was thrown out with the bathwater. As this book will show, psychotherapy has as strong a base in scientific evidence as any drug on the market. Newer forms of treatment, such as cognitive-behavioral therapy, have a solid base in science, but are most often provided by psychologists.

The force driving psychiatry today is its wish to be accepted as a medical specialty. To gain acceptance, psychiatry adopted a new paradigm paralleling the worldview of internal medicine, in which practice is based on systematic diagnosis, laboratory tests, and drug prescriptions. This change was overdue and was in most ways positive. But since our knowledge base remains sadly undeveloped, the idea that a new psychiatry can be built entirely on neuroscience is a dangerous illusion. In spite of all its advances, brain research has thus far taken only baby steps. It will be many decades before the complexity of the brain is unraveled and the true causes of mental disorders are known.

In reality, psychiatrists are treating conditions that they barely understand. Our diagnoses are, at best, rough and ready, and do not deserve the status of categories in other specialties. We have no laboratory tests that can reliably identify any mental disorder, and the measures we use are entirely based on clinical observations. Although our drugs can be powerful and effective (when used properly), we are over-prescribing them and offering them to patients who do not need them.

This book will challenge the myth of the expert who cures mental illnesses by adjusting and adding medications. Psychiatrists could help more people by spending less time with prescription pads and more time listening and talking to their patients. But this does not mean we should return to the analytic couch. It means, at least in part, that psychiatrists have to be interested in patients' lives and understand how events influence symptoms. They also need to acknowledge what they know and what they do not know so they can treat patients more intelligently and more effectively.

The Best of Both Worlds

This book will focus on the cost of psychiatry's shift in orientation. The choice of a narrowly medical identity that focuses exclusively on biological research and treatments has led to an impoverished practice. Biology is a necessary part of the theory and practice of psychiatry but does not provide a complete explanation of disease or a comprehensive guide to treatment. Psychiatrists diagnose patients from a manual and convince themselves that they are describing illnesses as specific as stroke or breast cancer. Even more seriously, some psychiatrists have forgotten how to talk to people. Many prescribe medication and do little else.

This critique should not in any way be seen as devaluing biological research or biological treatments. The conditions psychiatrists treat affect the brain. But this does not mean that the *source* of mental problems always lies at the level of neurons. Our psychological and social environment can make us anxious or depressed, leading in turn to changes in brain function. A discipline devoted to mental illness cannot ignore the mind.

The biological paradigm that dominates psychiatry today can be understood as a reaction *against* the past, when theories were spun out of thin air and patients were offered unscientific methods of treatment. But this book is not intended in any way to be an attack on psychiatry itself. We have had too much of that sort of thing. Starting with Thomas Szasz, "anti-psychiatrists" have refused to accept the biological basis of mental illness, and some even seem to think that psychiatrists should stop prescribing drugs (Breggin, 1994; Szasz, 1974). The very real benefits of pharmacological treatment would be lost if we were to adopt such backward-looking and misguided ideas. Psychiatrists must resist an either/or attitude when it comes to the study and treatment of mental illness.

Who This Book Is for and What It Is About

I have written this book for several audiences. Health professionals and trainees, inside or outside psychiatry, will want to know where the field is going and how much science is behind it. Moreover, since this book emphasizes the importance of scientific practice, I will be quoting data to support most of what I have to say. Of course, there are many controversies in psychiatry, and I do not have enough space to go into all of them in depth. And however much I am committed to evidence-based psychiatry, there are many important issues about which we have very limited data. But wherever I express a clinical opinion based on my own experience, I will make that clear.

I also hope that nonprofessionals will find this book enlightening. In an era of open information, psychiatric patients (and their families) need to understand the concepts behind our specialty. The educated public, which has long had a special interest in the field, needs to be updated on the vast changes occurring in psychiatry.

In summary, this book aims to provide an overview of contemporary psychiatry—how we got there, where we are now, and what is likely to happen in the future. As an academic, a researcher, and a teacher, I examine the discipline from the perspective of an insider. And as a practitioner who has always been committed to a psychiatry rooted in biology and psychology, I have written a book that aims to provide a balanced point of view, taking into account the strengths and weaknesses of both perspectives.

PART I

MODELS

1

Neuroscience and Psychiatry

Almost every day, one can read media reports on the latest developments in neuroscience. Scientific journals are packed with exciting
new findings. As a result, we have never known so much about the human
brain as we do now, and psychiatrists and their patients could eventually
be among the beneficiaries of this research. New research has, for example,
raised hope that the causes of mental illness will be explained by brain
abnormalities. It has also spurred investigations into genetics and specifically prompted a search for genes that may be associated with mental
disorders. Meanwhile, a large body of research has examined the role of
neurotransmitters in these disorders. Part of what has made this extraordinary brain science possible involves new imaging techniques that, by
producing dramatic pictures of the brain, seem to unlock its secrets. A
large body of research has examined how neurotransmitters are involved in
mental disorders. Even more exciting is the prospect that research in
neuroscience may lead to new and more effective methods of treatment.

The advances in neuroscience in recent years have, without doubt,
been scientifically impressive. But how do they affect medical practice?
Will the psychiatrist of tomorrow prescribe more powerful drugs guided

by gene profiles and brain scans? Will future psychiatrists become high-tech practitioners, differing little from specialists in internal medicine? Research leaders in psychiatry have little doubt that the field is headed precisely in that direction. They believe that most mental disorders are due to abnormal biology. Many psychiatrists have accepted this idea, and for them the primacy of neuroscience has become almost a dogma.

Is Psychiatry Different from Neurology?

In a 2005 article, "Psychiatry as a Clinical Neuroscience Discipline," published in the *Journal of the American Medical Association,* Thomas Insel (director of the National Institute of Mental Health) and Rémi Quirion (director of the Canadian Institute of Psychiatry and Neuro-sciences) argued that mental illnesses are complex genetic disorders in which abnormalities in brain chemistry and circuitry lead to behavioral symptoms (Insel & Quirion, 2005; for a similar view, see Martin, 2002). Insel, a psychiatrist best known for research on how brain hormones influence mating behavior in rodents, and Quirion, a PhD neuroscientist who studies brain chemistry, are influential administrators directing the future of psychiatric research. They acknowledge that mental disorders emerge from interactions between genetic predispositions and environ-mental stressors but recommend that psychiatry redefine itself as a form of "applied neuroscience."

This is a point of view that has captured psychiatry and that has critical implications for practice. If psychiatry is applied neuroscience, then drugs to restore normal brain chemistry would be the primary tool for the treatment of mental illness. Significantly, the words "psychology" and "psychotherapy" are not to be found anywhere in this article.

Insel and Quirion also suggested that the division between psychi-atry and neurology, which goes back to the 19th century, is artificial and unnecessary. They recommended that because both medical specialties treat diseases of the brain, they should be reunited into one discipline.

But why did psychiatry become separated from neurology in the first place? One reason is that mental disorders produce changes in thinking, emotion, and behavior; neurological disorders, although they can pro-duce mental effects similar to those seen in diseases treated by psychi-atrists, primarily concern physical symptoms (such as paralysis, abnormal movements, or loss of sensation).

Another reason for the separation was that neurological diseases (like strokes or multiple sclerosis) cause visible damage to the brain. Neurologists can explain symptoms on the basis of which structures of the brain are affected. In the past, no one was able to locate any form of brain damage in diseases of the mind (like schizophrenia).

Recent research has challenged this division. More subtle effects on brain anatomy and physiology can now be measured, and imaging studies show that specific regions can "light up" differently in specific mental disorders. In the past, when an organic cause was found for diseases formerly seen as "psychiatric" (such as tertiary syphilis), the diseases were transferred to neurology (Shorter, 1997). The argument can be made that the same process will happen with schizophrenia and mood disorders once their effects on the brain are properly mapped. In this context, one might readily imagine a future in which all brain diseases are treated by one specialty.

A few of the more severe disorders psychiatrists treat, including schizophrenia, melancholic depression, and bipolar disorder, may not actually be different from neurological conditions. These are disorders in which the evidence for brain abnormalities is strong, and in which the environment plays a relatively minor role. These are the diseases in which biological therapies are the most useful.

However, most of the disorders that psychiatrists see do not fit into this model. To reduce most cases of depression, anxiety, eating disorders, or personality disorder to brain damage would be rather simplistic. As later chapters in this book will show, understanding these conditions requires a model that takes life circumstances into account, even for the so-called biologically caused mental illnesses like schizophrenia.

A narrowly biological view to treatment runs counter to the approach that has characterized psychiatry for decades. A *biopsychosocial* model of mental illness, in which disorders are seen as arising from interactions between biological, psychological, and social factors, was proposed by the American psychiatrist George Engel (Engel, 1980). This model has been highly influential and emphasizes interfaces between psychiatry and other disciplines—not only neuroscience but psychology and other social sciences as well. Psychiatrists who use a broad theory are more likely to offer a broad range of treatments, including psychotherapy and social interventions.

Turning psychiatry into applied neuroscience would strip psychiatry of much of what makes it unique. It would also support a style of practice in which the main thing that psychiatrists do is prescribe drugs. If psychiatry becomes "mindless" and consists of nothing more than the clinical application of neuroscience, patient care will suffer.

To adapt a famous quotation from the Vietnam War, Insel and Quirion seem to believe it is necessary to destroy psychiatry in order to save it. They propose a model in which the main skill of psychiatrists is knowing how to repair twisted molecules. But psychiatry is a humanistic medical discipline, not a branch of chemistry. Moreover, recombining psychiatry and neurology into one specialty would not make sense as long as psychiatrists continue to see patients with psychological problems. And finally, after a hundred years of separation, each specialty has its own traditions and its own culture. Neurology, for example, has always taken pride in its ability to explain disease by precise effects on sites in the brain (or in peripheral nerves). Its patients are treated with drugs or surgery. Most of its practitioners know little about depression, do not recognize it or find it interesting, and hardly ever treat it. If they do recognize symptoms of a mental health condition in their patients with, say, Parkinson's disease or multiple sclerosis, they are likely to consult a psychiatrist about the ideal treatment for those symptoms.

Causes and Risk Factors

What causes mental illness? By and large, advances in neuroscience notwithstanding, we still don't know. But as human beings, psychiatrists are not immune to the temptation to believe that in fact they have the answers to these unanswered questions. And as practitioners who are trained to heal and who daily face enormous human suffering, they are not the type of people who can afford to be paralyzed by doubt.

The problem is that there is no one answer to the question of what causes mental illness. Most illnesses do not have simple or single causes. With the exception of a few genetic diseases, pathology arises from the interaction of many factors (Paris, 1999). Some are hereditary, whereas others are environmental. Each factor, by itself, contributes to the overall risk. But no single risk is the cause of any one disease. What best predicts illness is the total weight of all risk factors. This model is called *stress-diathesis theory* (Monroe & Simons, 1991). The idea behind the model is that people do not fall ill from stress unless they are vulnerable (i.e., have a diathesis), and those who have a diathesis will not fall ill unless they are stressed. Only when the weight of risk factors exceeds the threshold of the patient's vulnerability does overt illness emerge.

Failure to consider this complexity can lead to wrong conclusions. Thus, when research demonstrates a statistical relationship between a risk and a disease, we may be tempted to conclude that one is the cause of the other. Yet even when a strong relationship is found, causality is not proven. For example, data may show that risk and disease are correlated in a large number of cases, but the confluence may occur only in a minority. Thus, most people with the disease will not have the risk, and most people with the risk will not develop the disease.

This mistake has also afflicted past psychological theories of mental illness. For example, a number of mental disorders are associated with childhood trauma and family dysfunction (Paris, 1999). However, it does not follow that all our patients must have had an unhappy childhood. Many will have had a childhood no worse than anyone else's. Statistical relationships arise because some patients (and not all) are particularly sensitive to stressful events because of their temperamental vulnerabilities.

What research has demonstrated (but not everyone knows) is that most people who suffer childhood trauma and family dysfunction function normally as adults (Paris, 2000a). A large degree of resilience has been repeatedly shown in community surveys of people exposed to adverse events (Rutter & Rutter, 1993). In the face of trauma, even the worst kind, the vast majority of people never develop posttraumatic stress disorder (McFarlane, 1989; McNally, 1999). Most people are resilient to stress. If they were not, the human species would have gone extinct long ago.

Neuroscientists who account for mental disorders entirely through biological correlates are making a mistake similar to that of their psychotherapeutic predecessors. Again, one can see strong associations between a biological marker, such as a gene or a change in a brain structure, and a mental illness. But this need not mean that every case of the disease will be associated with the marker—research usually shows that most are not. Nor does it mean that everyone who has the marker will get the disease—most will not.

One can identify several reasons for the discrepancy. First, with a few exceptions, no single biological risk factor leads predictably to disease. Thus, even in mental disorders with strong genetic components, such as schizophrenia or bipolar illness, no *single* gene is associated with illness (Braff, Freedman, Schork, & Gottesman, 2007a). Instead, one sees a pattern of *complex inheritance* in which many genes in combination (we are not sure exactly how many) produce vulnerability (van den Bree & Owen, 2003; Prathikanti & Weinberger, 2005). It requires a complex genetic mix to produce susceptibility to mental disorders.

Second, genes associated with illness may never be expressed unless the individual is placed in a specific environment. A new science of *epigenetics* (the study of heritable traits that do not involve changes to the underlying DNA sequence) examines how genes can be "turned on" or "turned off" by the environment (Petronis et al., 2000). Genetic variations can be positive, negative, or neutral, depending on environmental context. A large body of research shows that people are most likely to develop mental disorders when they are genetically vulnerable *and* exposed to a stressful life situation (Caspi et al., 2002, 2003).

Third, the diseases psychiatrists treat are not well defined. Scientists refer to this as "the phenotype problem," where one cannot identify genetic vulnerability (*genotype*) associated with disease without first establishing how they are expressed in thought, emotion, and behavior (*phenotype*) (Flint & Munafo, 2007). Moreover, visible phenotypes reflect underlying biological processes referred to as *endophenotypes*. As we will see, some of the categories of illness used in psychiatry are so broad and fuzzy that studying their biological markers with any specificity is an almost hopeless task. If we were to break larger categories down into more specific entities, they might have more specific correlates.

One of the great mysteries of psychiatry is the fact that many people with severe mental disorders are fairly normal up to the age when they fall ill. Quite a few mental disorders begin in adolescence after a normal childhood—some young people who develop schizophrenia have functioned reasonably well until a few years before the illness starts (van Nimwegen, de Haan, van Beveren, van den Brink, & Linszen, 2005). This observation points to the importance of brain development and the role of environmental stressors in precipitating illness. We are all born with vulnerabilities, yet most of us never become ill.

Genes and biological markers are linked to variations in temperament (Nigg, 2006; Rutter, Moffit, & Caspi, 2006). *Temperament* refers to individual differences in behavior that are present at birth. But temperamental differences do not produce mental illness. Simply put, we are all different. Some of us are shy, others bold. Some are emotional, others stoic. These characteristics all have a biological component and can, under certain conditions, be associated with a risk for a mental disorder. However, all these temperamental patterns are compatible with normality.

In summary, there is no direct cause-and-effect relationship between either biological or psychological factors and mental disorders. The overall risk for disorder is cumulative (Rutter & Rutter, 1993). People become ill only when they suffer from temperamental vulnerability *and* are exposed to environmental stressors. This is why no theory exclusively based on biology (or psychology) can explain why people develop mental illness.

How Well Does Neuroscience Explain Mental Illness?

A careful look at the relevance of neuroscience for psychiatry uncovers a more humbling picture than is often drawn in current scientific literature. Research in neuroscience is still in its infancy. In spite of recent triumphs, we still know little about how the brain works. Future generations could think of contemporary neuroscience the way we see Columbus's voyages to America—he made a courageous exploration but lacked a good map.

The problem might be understood by comparing the brain to the heart or kidney. Instead of a muscular pump or filtration system, we are looking at a network of billions of neurons, capable of producing consciousness, free will, and highly complex behaviors. It took many decades to understand hearts and kidneys. For the brain, the time line will be much longer. It will be longer still before our knowledge of the brain translates into a deeper understanding of the mind and of all that can go wrong with it, as in mental illness.

Later in this chapter, we will consider what genes, imaging, and neurochemistry tell us about mental illness now. Broadly speaking, we live in an era where DNA has become an icon of science. Yet genes lack consistent associations with major mental illnesses. Positron emission tomography (PET) scans and magnetic resonance imaging (MRI) produce beautiful pictures. Everyone has seen them—they show areas of the brain "lighting up," as if we were visualizing the very chemistry of thought. (Actually, the brilliant colors of brain scans are added artificially.) Yet while imaging suggests that disorders affect specific parts of the brain, they have explained little about the *causes* of most forms of mental illness. Finally, research on communication through neurotransmitters, and on chemical processes within neurons, is impressive. But these findings have also not shed great light on the causes of mental illness.

Psychiatrists are hoping that breakthroughs in neuroscience will lead to improved treatment for patients. Paradoxically, the great breakthroughs in psychopharmacology occurred decades ago, before any of the mechanisms by which drugs worked had even been discovered. If psychiatrists were to prescribe in much the same way they did a generation ago, their patients might not notice a great difference.

Fifty years ago, when I was an undergraduate student, little was known about the brain. No neurotransmitters had been definitively identified. The only form of imaging available was a skull X-ray. The brain was a kind of "black box," most of whose regions appeared to have no specific function.

While neuroscience has greatly advanced since then, progress should not blind us to our still vast ignorance about the human brain. As Isaac Newton once remarked about his own discoveries, "I feel like a child who while playing by the seashore has found a few bright colored shells and a few pebbles while the whole vast ocean of truth stretches out almost untouched and unruffled before my eager fingers."[1] The same can be said about our limited knowledge of the brain. An extremely complex structure, it has billions of cells that can be connected in billions of ways. Each of these cells is—to shift to a different metaphor now—a factory producing proteins under the guidance of half of all the genes in the human genome (Andreasen, 2001). A great deal can and does go awry in this system, and in ways that we largely do not yet understand.

Reductionism and Emergence

The question of whether neuroscience can be the primary basis of psychiatry should be seen in the context of two larger questions. The *mind-brain problem* concerns whether the mind and its thought are equivalent to (and determined by) activity in the brain (Schimmel, 2001a, 2001b). This is a philosophical issue, and most psychiatrists do not usually get involved in philosophy (even the philosophy of science). Nonetheless, what one believes about the question has a vast impact on clinical practice and on the direction of psychiatry.

The mind-brain problem might conceivably be resolved through empirical data. For now, many philosophers and neuroscientists have weighed in on the question. Whereas some claim that mental processes and human consciousness are ultimately an illusion and that the only reality is the physics, chemistry, and biology of neurons (Churchland, 1995), others insist that thought and consciousness exist in their own right and that the mind can determine (through its capacity for "free will") what happens in the brain (Searle, 2004).

A broader question concerns whether larger-scale phenomena in nature can be explained by small-scale phenomena. This approach, called *reductionism,* has been applied to the study of the mind, explaining complex phenomena like the human brain through simpler mechanisms, "reducing" mind to the actions of neurons, chemical transmitters, and specific proteins (Jones, 2000). This approach leads to the idea that illnesses with behavioral symptoms can be explained entirely through brain mechanisms. In other words, behind every twisted thought must be a twisted molecule.

Reductionism is a strategy with a long history of success. Over the centuries, science has triumphed by reducing the large to the small, and the complex to the simple. Different levels of science can be linked in this way. Physics studies matter by breaking it down into atoms, and nuclear physics has broken down the atom—first into particles, then into quarks. Chemistry was linked to physics through Mendeleev's periodic table, which showed that all molecules are combinations of only 92 natural elements. Biology has been linked to chemistry through the discovery that living organisms make use of molecules to perform many functions. And psychology has been linked to biology by research showing that changes in the brain can influence behavior.

Although many scientific advances have resulted from reductionism, the approach has definite limits (Jones, 2000). Some observations are illuminated by mechanisms at a simpler level, but not everything is explained. The whole is usually more than the sum of its parts, and larger-scale phenomena usually need to be studied in their own right. For example, the reality of a table cannot be accounted for by atoms and quarks. The properties of hydrogen and oxygen do not explain the molecular characteristics of water. Biological organisms are not robots driven by chemistry and physiology. And even though molecules are necessary for consciousness, they do not explain it.

Psychiatry, which treats and studies the mind, faces a more complex reality than do other specialties. Medicine may have gone mad over molecules, but livers, brains, and kidneys have no will of their own. One does not have to be a dualist (or believe in a soul) to consider the mind a subject of independent study (Jones, 2000). Mental processes cannot exist without a functioning brain. But it is a logical error to conclude that all pathways of causation must go "upward," from neurons to mental processes. Causation can also go "downward," from cellular structures to genes and proteins (Noble, 2006), as well as from thought to behavior (i.e., the existence of "free will").

Needless to say, not everyone agrees with this point of view. It has been argued repeatedly that consciousness and free will are illusions (Dennett, 1991). But even if they were, we would still need to study the mind on its own terms. To prove that reductionism works, one would have to show that complex forms of behavior can be predicted from biology alone. Neuroscience is nowhere near such a goal. It is replete with associations, and short on predictions.

Mental processes are influenced by multiple factors, only some of which can be understood at the level of molecules. The mind, with its crucial (although still unexplained) property of consciousness, operates at a different level. This idea is not "holistic" mush but follows directly from the nature of complex phenomena. Although mind cannot exist without brain, it represents another level of analysis—one with features that cannot be fully explained at the level of neurons.

Models of complexity, such as "general systems theory," suggest that systems have *emergent* properties that cannot be explained by their components (von Bertalanffy, 1968). Emergence is defined as a process in which complex *patterns* arise from simpler components and in which higher-level patterns are unpredictable from phenomena at a lower level (Beckermann, Flohr, & Kim, 1992).

A good example in modern science is the relationship between the structure of DNA and the development of organisms. DNA does not determine how the body develops. It is a recipe, not a blueprint. Just as making a cake from a recipe will not always produce the same result because of varying circumstances, the environment (which turns genes on and off) makes everyone different. (This is why even identical twins do not have the same traits.) The new science of epigenetics, focusing on the interactions between genes and environment, may help us understand these complexities (Meaney & Szyf, 2005). Consider the following example. The conscious mind arises from the interactions of billions of neurons in the human brain. Yet no single neuron is capable of thought. That is what is meant by emergence. When we study complex phenomena such as human behavior, we have to reverse the process of reductionism and practice integration, that is, study complex phenomena on their own terms while not ignoring links to other levels of analyses. Reductionism is a powerful tool that should not be discarded and will continue to play a role in psychiatric research. (In fact, Chapter 3 suggests that psychiatric diagnoses will never be valid without using biological markers that have proved so valuable in other areas of medicine.) Knowledge of brain mechanisms could also allow pharmacologists to develop new and more effective drugs.

Even so, psychiatrists should not set their sights on a utopian future in which neuroscience will solve most clinical problems. The science behind psychiatry needs a broader and more comprehensive framework. Clinical symptoms such as pain are features of consciousness. In the same way, depression is an emergent property of the mind.

I recently attended a conference in which basic neuroscientists described how their skills might be applied to mental disorders. One researcher working on neural growth suggested that he might be able to solve the problem of schizophrenia if someone could define an abnormal protein that would be a phenotype for the illness. But that is just what psychiatry cannot do!

Nonetheless, the best research has the capacity to establish a link between the complex and the simple. Cognitive neuroscience differs from classical neuroscience in that it concerns thought and not just neurotransmitter activity (Pinker, 1997). This new and productive field examines relationships between various types of thinking processes and activity in specific brain structures. It takes the mind seriously, and although cognitive scientists are deeply interested in the brain mechanisms behind thought, they study mental processes on their own terms.

In summary, reductionism is a philosophical principle but is not "just philosophy." This is a point of view that underlies the current impoverishment of the practice of psychiatry. If you believe that depression consists of nothing but disordered neurotransmitters and that life circumstances affecting mood are not particularly relevant, you do not really need to learn how to talk to people. You just need to reach for your prescription pad and correct the chemistry.

Genetics

That psychiatrists have learned a great deal about the brain from research in neuroscience is clear. (For a brief review of the principles of psychiatric genetics, see Prathikanti & Weinberger, 2005.) And the future of medicine as a whole will be influenced by what we know about genes. However, it is important to take a closer look at genetics to determine what it does and does not tell us now about disease.

The discovery of DNA was followed by the deciphering of the genetic code, showing how this molecule guides the construction of proteins—the building blocks of all organisms. More recently, the sequencing of the human genome revealed a surprise—we manage with only 20,000-plus genes—not much more than many less intelligent creatures. Thus the complexity of the human body is not built on the total number of genes but how they are used. About half are involved in building the brain. Given that the absolute number of neurons in the human brain is about one trillion and that neurons are widely interconnected, their potential combinations could number more than all the stars in the universe.

Physicians, scientists, and the educated public are awaiting the therapeutic breakthroughs expected to follow inevitably from genetic discoveries. At a minimum, patients in the future could have their genomes scanned to find out which disease they are most susceptible to. At a maximum, gene therapy could be used to reverse the course of diseases.

Yet the hard facts are that we are nowhere near any of these goals. To understand why, consider how genes actually work. First, genes make proteins, not diseases. Even if we were able to identify all human genes, we would still need to know what proteins they make. The emerging science of "proteomics" aims to do just that—to reduce all biological processes to protein synthesis. (For a review of proteomics, see Twyman, 2004.) But it will take decades to accomplish this.

Second, when genes do affect susceptibility to disease, complex inheritance is the rule, not the exception. For this reason, there is no such thing as a gene "for" most of the diseases in medicine, and it is rare for single genes to be associated with specific diagnoses (Kendler, 2006). A Mendelian scenario (named after Gregor Mendel, the founder of scientific genetics) occurs only in a few rare conditions. Most of the illnesses that physicians treat do not develop in this way. In the most common human diseases (such as arteriosclerosis and cancer), associations with single genes that have been identified account for more than a small percentage of the total variance. Disease susceptibility could be associated with variations in as many as 20 or 30 genes in various combinations.

Third, genes are "turned off" most of the time (Meaney & Szyf, 2005). To become active, they must interact with the environment. (A genetic susceptibility to lung cancer, for example, may never show itself clinically unless the patient also smokes.)

Fourth, even when genes associated with disease can be identified, applying this knowledge in a practical way is not easy. A decade after a gene strongly associated with cystic fibrosis was discovered, for example, patients suffering from this terrible disease have not yet benefited (Rosenhecker, Huth, & Rudolph, 2006).

In short, although genetic knowledge will *eventually* benefit psychiatry, we are decades away from practical application. Moreover, since mental disorders are based on complex genetic dispositions subject to environmental influences, the study of single genes will probably not help psychiatrists treat patients. This is not to say that genetics is not of importance to psychiatry—it could turn out to have supreme importance. But genes are only one piece of a much more complex puzzle.

Imaging

Specialists in other areas of medicine have long been able to "see" the organs in which disease occurs, by feeling them through the skin, observing them during surgical operations, or using advanced radiological techniques. One of the great frustrations for psychiatrists has been that they cannot observe the brains of people with mental disorders but instead must rely on observable or self-reported signs and symptoms in order to assess what their patients are experiencing. With the arrival of new imaging technology, however, psychiatrists now have several methods for "seeing" inside the brain and observing its activity (Morihisa, 2001).

In the 1970s, computerized tomography (CT) scans began to replace X-rays as a way to visualize the brain. These impressive machines yielded unparalleled pictures that looked like slices of the brain, with a readily visible and detailed structure. Although these images told us little about function, CT scans were striking enough to be used in court cases in which the presence of mental illness was an issue (as happened in the case of John Hinckley, discussed in Chapter 12).

Magnetic resonance imaging (MRI) provided even better pictures of brain slices, and the development of functional imaging was even more of a breakthrough. Functional MRI (fMRI) allows researchers to examine patients' brains while the patients are performing tasks or experiencing emotions. This technique is easier to administer and gives a more precise image. In positive emission tomography (PET), the patient is injected with a radioactive isotope that resembles chemicals used in specific areas of the brain and not in others. The beauty of the pictures produced by these scans is that one can see brain areas "lighting up" in association with a specific function. As a result, we now have much more information about which brain regions do what.

These methods have greatly illuminated research in neuroscience. Seeing what parts of the brain become active in relation to thought, emotion, and behavior is of enormous significance. However, localized brain activity is just as likely to be a result of mental activity as it is to be a cause of it. Thus far, imaging has had few clinical applications to diseases like schizophrenia or mood disorders (Nemeroff, Kilts, & Berns, 1999). That situation could change in the future, but at this point practical use of imaging to guide treatment remains only a hope.

Neurotransmitters

Fifty years ago we knew little about how neurons communicate with each other. It was thought that electric sparks jumped the gap between the end of one neuron and the beginning of another. Today, we know that neurotransmission, while partly electrical, mainly depends on a large number of chemical messengers, many of which are simple molecules (others are proteins). Neurons have different receptors for these chemicals, so the same transmitters produce different effects at different sites. All these events take place at the junction between one neuron and another—the synapse.

Molecules derived from the amino acids in our diet do much of the work. One is glutamate, the most widely distributed of all neurotransmitters, which excites neurons beyond the synapse. Another is gamma-amino butyric acid (GABA), an amino acid that functions as the main inhibitory transmitter in the brain.

The most studied group of neurotransmitters for psychiatry is the *monoamines*, a group of molecules derived from amino acids that are produced in older, deeper structures of the brain. These chemicals mainly act to modulate the effect of other transmitters higher up in the brain (Nestler, Hyman, & Malenka, 2001).

One monoamine is dopamine, a substance thought to be particularly important for addictions because it is concentrated in brain systems involved in pleasure or emotional reward (Schultz, 2006). Because some antipsychotic drugs block the action of dopamine, a long-standing theory in psychiatry has proposed that schizophrenia results from abnormalities in receptors for this transmitter. This theory was, in the end, not supported by sufficient evidence, and current research on schizophrenia focuses more on glutamate (Coyle, 2006).

Norepinephrine, a neurotransmitter associated with stress responses, activates many brain systems and the sympathetic nervous system. Several antidepressant drugs increase the activity of this transmitter through their effects on receptors at synapses. However, this theory of antidepressant action, once dominant in psychiatry, turned out to be too simple (Iversen, 2006).

Serotonin has been the most important of all neurotransmitters in psychiatric research. This substance has very broad effects on the brain and is particularly important for its relationship to depression, anxiety, and impulsivity (Carver & Miller, 2006). The theory that serotonin is deficient in many mental disorders has long been current, although research has failed to find any consistent deficiency of this kind (Valenstein, 1998). However, antidepressants cause neurons to keep serotonin around longer at the synapse, which has been hypothesized to be one of the mechanisms of their effect.

Unlike genes and neuroimaging, research on neurotransmitters has had practical applications in the treatment of mental disorders. For example, SSRIs were developed as "designer drugs" for increasing serotonin activity at the synapse (Kramer, 1993). Yet for many of the drugs that psychiatrists prescribe, the reasons for their effectiveness remain unknown. After fifty years, psychiatrists still do not understand why antipsychotic drugs help patients with schizophrenia, how lithium and other mood stabilizers help control bipolar disorder, or what precise effects antidepressants have on neurotransmitters.

One reason for this uncertainty is that drugs affect several chemical systems, not just one (see Schatzberg & Nemeroff, 2004). Another major unsolved mystery concerns why antidepressants take several weeks to be fully effective in many patients. One possibility is that they encourage neurons to grow new connections, which takes time.

In summary, although research on neurotransmitters has had a strong relationship to drug development, we are left with more questions than answers. These chemicals have different effects in different parts of the brain, which is not just a "soup" of chemicals but a complex organ with a structure and a physiology.

Neural Networks

The brain operates through connections among billions of neurons. But for a long time the function of large areas of the brain remained a mystery. We have long known the location of sensory and motor areas in the brain, but much of the cerebral cortex (the part that thinks) was unmapped.

Imaging studies have helped unlock this mystery (Mandzia & Black, 2001). For example, we now know that the prefrontal and orbital cortexes, regions of the brain that lie at the front of the head and behind the eyes, have a special role in decision making and controlling impulsivity. We can also distinguish among parts of the cortex that affect specific aspects of thought. For example, the anterior cingulate gyrus, a structure lying deeper in the brain, has roles in decision making, attention, and memory. Deep inside the temporal lobe of the brain are the hippocampus, the main center for short-term memory, and the amygdala, a region governing responses associated with fear and unexpected events.

These discoveries have led to research—much of it using PET and fMRI—in which brain structures are examined to see whether they function differently in mental disorders. In many cases, they do. Yet again, such observations do not tell us why. Are we looking at causes or effects? This growing area of neuroscience is still in its infancy.

Conclusion

For all that it has accomplished, neuroscience has not yet delivered a convincing understanding of the causes of mental disorders. One can hardly compare our knowledge of the brain to what we know about the heart or the kidney and their diseases. But to dismiss the dramatic advances in neuroscience would be foolish. Every year our knowledge of the brain grows by leaps and bounds. And what has been discovered so far is only the beginning.

One might say that neuroscience is still awaiting its Newton—that is, someone who can produce a theory that will make sense out of complexity. It might take fifty to a hundred years for that to happen. In the meantime, one can practice psychiatry and help most of one's patients without knowing precisely how the brain works.

But there is a more immediate issue. In principle, nothing in neuroscience prevents clinicians from being empathic and interested in the lives of their patients and from trying to understand their difficulties in the context of their total experience. This is the essence of the biopsychosocial perspective, and the best psychiatrists, whatever their orientation, do try to bring this perspective into their work. However, we need only to look around us to see the clinical results of the current obsession with the neurobiology of mental illness—and the many psychiatrists giving out prescriptions without taking the time to understand the specific problems that affect patients. Even if a working knowledge of neuroscience is an essential part of psychiatric practice, it does not fully explain the mind—or provide the whole answer to treating mental illness.

2

Psychotherapy and Psychiatry

In the 1960s, when I trained to be a psychiatrist, I expected to spend most of my career sitting in an armchair conducting psychotherapy. Many young doctors in my generation had the same idea. Psychotherapy was what attracted us to psychiatry. We were idealistic young doctors who wanted to work with people. The attraction to psychiatry was so powerful that 40 years ago up to 10% of medical students went into psychiatry. Only 2–3% make that choice today. (For a recent review, see Sierles et al., 2003.)

While most psychiatrists do still try to talk meaningfully to their patients, they have less curiosity about the inner recesses of the mind and are no longer trained to be empathic. A prominent research psychologist recently said to me, "You have to assume that psychiatrists under the age of 40 are just not interested in therapy." What they are mainly interested in instead is expert skills in pharmacology.

This dramatic change in psychiatry's identity has affected the kinds of treatment that patients receive. Psychotherapy, once the central tool of our profession, has become a marginal aspect of our work. Paradoxically, this change occurred at a time when research definitively proved that psychotherapies are effective.

This chapter will review the scientific status of modern psychotherapy and discuss *why* and *how* it works. I will then examine the psychological theories of mental disorders that underlie the classical talk therapies, explain why they are out of date, and suggest how they need to be modified.

Eysenck's Challenge

Fifty years ago, psychoanalysis held a prominent place on both sides of the Atlantic, yet researchers had never examined its effectiveness. Then the British psychologist Hans Eysenck (1916–1997), an iconoclast with little patience for conventional wisdom, came along to issue a provocative challenge. In 1952 he published an article in the *Journal of Consulting Psychology* entitled "The Effects of Psychotherapy: An Evaluation." In this often-cited paper, he pointed out that in spite of there being a large clinical literature on traditional talk therapies, such as psychoanalytically based forms of therapy, no one had ever proven that these methods actually work.

Physicians expect drugs to be tested in clinical trials, and psychotherapy can and should be assessed in the same way. Such research usually involves comparing the effects of a treatment to a placebo or to no treatment. When Eysenck compared the claimed effectiveness of psychotherapy to the effectiveness of no treatment, he showed that active treatment had little advantage over watchful waiting. Eysenck later became involved in the development of behavior therapy, a method he believed could succeed where traditional methods had failed.

Although Eysenck's challenge was not really based on systematic data, it had an explosive impact—at first, all one heard were howls of outrage. Psychoanalysts who lacked scientific training but who "knew" that their treatment worked dismissed his criticisms. But as psychology became more scientifically rigorous, researchers accepted the challenge to prove whether talk therapies work. Eysenck's article ultimately had a positive effect because it prompted many studies seeking to examine the questions he raised.

By 1978 psychotherapy research literature was strong enough for a large book to be written summarizing what clinical trials had shown. That volume, edited by two leading researchers in the field, Allen E. Bergin and Sol S. Garfield, was the *Handbook of Psychotherapy and Behavior Change* (which has since been revised about every seven years) (Lambert, 2003). Still considered the "bible" of psychotherapy research, the fifth edition of this handbook, now edited by Michael Lambert of Brigham Young University, follows the tradition of its previous editions and summarizes the enormous body of data that has accumulated on the topic. As we will see, the data not only indicates that talk therapies *do* work, but it also shows *how* they work. Let us review these results.

What Psychotherapy Research Shows

Fifty years after Eysenck's challenge, there can be no further doubt that psychotherapy is more effective (for most patients) than naturalistic recovery without treatment. As an influential 1980 book integrating the literature states, "Psychotherapy benefits people of all ages as reliably as school educates them, medicine cures them, or business turns a profit" (Smith, Glass, & Miller, 1980, p. 10). Nothing in the last quarter century has emerged to change that verdict.

This does not mean that *everyone* benefits from psychotherapy. As is the case with the use of most psychiatric drugs, some people receiving psychotherapy recover completely, others improve, and some fail to benefit at all. Yet in the aggregate, psychotherapy works much better than no treatment at all.

We know this to be so from the results of hundreds of published clinical trials. These studies can be combined to calculate an overall effect (the technical term is "meta-analysis"), and their results show that psychological treatment is effective for the problems that most patients present with—that is, anxiety and depression—and for difficulties in work and relationships. The overall difference between treatment and no treatment can be described as an "effect size" of 0.8 (nearly one standard deviation, comparable to the difference between bright people and people of only average intelligence) (Lambert 2003; Smith et al., 1980, p. 10). Furthermore, psychotherapy helps most people who seek it, and its effects are often lasting.

There are two ways to study the effects of psychotherapy. One is *effectiveness* research, the study of treatment in naturalistic populations. The best-known example of this approach is a survey conducted by Martin Seligman of the University of Pennsylvania, derived from data obtained from thousands of readers of the magazine *Consumer Reports* (Seligman, 1995). The study asked its subjects to describe their experiences with psychotherapy and to what extent they had benefited from it.

There is value in studying psychotherapy in a "naturalistic" way, that is, in the real world rather than in an experiment. However, the problem with that type of research is that it fails to use a *control group*. Would patients have gotten well with a different type of treatment, or no treatment at all? The *Consumer Reports* survey could not answer that question. We also do not know whether the readers of that magazine (highly educated, committed to quality, and self-selected by answering the survey) were representative of the larger population of therapy patients.

The second and more precise approach to studying psychotherapy is to examine its effects in the same way that we test drugs. This is called *efficacy* research, the study of treatment in controlled trials, in which patients are assigned randomly to a treatment (i.e., treatment versus no treatment, or treatment versus a form of minimal support). The main problem with interpreting randomized controlled trials (RCTs) is that of generalizing their results to patients seen in practice. People who enter clinical trials and agree to be randomized do not necessarily resemble the patients therapists see.

Thus, efficacy and effectiveness research present a kind of trade-off (Hogarty, Schooler, & Baker, 1997). Efficacy is based on a controlled experiment but may not be applicable to real patients; effectiveness is based on real-world data, but its lack of controls makes its results difficult to interpret. Still, in both methods we need to have a way to measure outcome; for example, we might rate changes in symptoms and assess quality of life (how patients function in work and relationships). And by and large, both approaches have produced evidence that therapy often not only helps reduce symptoms but also helps patients work more effectively and get along better with other people.

How does psychotherapy stack up against drugs? Researchers have conducted head-to-head comparisons of medication and therapy for similar conditions. In mild to moderate depression, talk therapy is just as effective as any antidepressant, but drugs or electroconvulsive therapy (ECT) are better for severe depression (Elkin, Shea, Watkins, & Imber, 1989). Yet in some conditions, psychotherapy produces unique effects based on specific methods (Lambert, 2003). For example, cognitive-behavioral psychotherapy has been shown to be specifically (if far from universally) effective in treating anxiety disorders (e.g., panic attacks, obsessions, and compulsions) (Butler, Chapman, Forman, & Beck, 2006). There are other diagnoses for which therapy has been shown more effective than drugs. This is the case for personality disorders, conditions in which the main problems are relationships with other people (Shea et al., 1990; Paris, 2003).

This data also shows that although most patients with psychological problems can benefit from taking medication, many will get better with talk therapy alone. By and large, medication is most essential for sicker patients—one cannot treat schizophrenia, severe and incapacitating depressions, or bipolar disorder without drugs. But even in these severely ill patients, researchers have shown that psychotherapy adds value to medication regimes (Tarrier, 2005).

How Psychotherapy Works

Jerome Frank (1909–2005) was a Johns Hopkins psychiatrist who also had a PhD in psychology—a fact that helps explain his strong commitment to science. Frank's ideas were far ahead of their time. His famous book *Persuasion and Healing* was published in 1962, when there was still little formal research in psychotherapy (Frank & Frank, 1991). In it, Frank provided a model that explains why many types of therapy work, independent of theories underlying specific methods.

Frank saw psychotherapy as a process in which patients arrive demoralized and hopeless but improve by regaining morale and hope. In his view, the *process* of the treatment is more important than what is said in the therapy room. Thus, psychotherapy is not a technical procedure but a healing relationship. Frank's conclusion was that the ideas behind different forms of therapy are largely irrelevant (he suggested that almost any theory will do if the patient is willing to accept it). Iconoclastically, Frank noted that traditional and faith healers have also had a fair record of success in managing psychological symptoms.

Over the next forty years, research has consistently supported Frank's position. The most striking confirmation comes in the form of *comparative trials* of psychotherapy. In this type of research, researchers randomly assign patients to different methods to see if one is better than another. It has consistently been found that no particular form of treatment is more effective than any other.

Lester Luborsky, a psychologist (and psychoanalyst) working at the University of Pennsylvania, is one of the deans of psychotherapy research. In 1975 Luborsky and his colleagues published a much-quoted paper entitled "Comparative Studies of Psychotherapy: Is It True That Everyone Has Won and All Shall Have Prizes?" The title echoed a 1936 paper by the psychology professor Saul Rosenzweig (1907–2004) (Duncan, 2002). Referring to the absence of differences in the outcome of various forms of psychotherapy, Rosenzweig, citing Lewis Carroll's *Alice in Wonderland* (in which the dodo declares after a race that everyone has won and all shall have prizes), wittily described the result as a "dodo bird" verdict.

Bruce Wampold, a psychologist at the University of Wisconsin, systematically reviewed the recent literature and concluded that a dodo-bird verdict for comparative trials still held (Wampold, 2001). When researchers compare one therapy to another, hardly any differences emerge. If technique is not that crucial, then the overall skill of the therapist in getting patients engaged in the process may be more important.

However, therapist skill may be as much a natural talent as something that can be learned. This conclusion is supported by research showing that experienced therapists are sometimes no more effective than novices. In a famous study in the 1970s at Vanderbilt University, Hans Strupp (1993) set out to demonstrate the importance of technique and experience. His research design compared the effectiveness of treatment from experienced therapists (including psychoanalysts) with that of "treatment" provided by university professors who had been rated by their students as being unusually sympathetic: No difference in outcome was found between patients seeing experienced therapists and those seeing novices. The limitation of the experiment was that the people receiving therapy were volunteers, not real patients with diagnosable problems. But the finding that therapeutic skills depend largely on a talent for empathy—the ability to connect with and ally oneself well with patients—rather than on experience has since been confirmed in many other studies (Lambert, 2003). One can conclude only that common factors (also called "nonspecific factors") in therapy are the best predictors of results, with the most important factor being *the quality of the alliance* between the therapist and the patient.

Jerome Frank had emphasized that therapy is a relationship and that psychotherapy provides troubled people with an "expert companion" who understands their distress and guides them out of a morass. Patients usually agree with that judgment. Instead of telling their friends how brilliant their therapist's comments are, they tell them how well they feel the therapist understands them. This is precisely what Hans Strupp and his colleagues (1969) discovered when they asked a group of patients what they got out of therapy: Most said they could not even remember what they had talked about—it was the process that felt good.

Other studies of the "therapeutic alliance," a measure of how well patient and therapist are working together, further support the importance of common factors in the success of a therapy (Luborsky & Luborsky, 2006). When researchers examine the course of therapy, they can often predict how the treatment will turn out after a few meetings. They do this by asking patients how they feel about the therapy and the therapist, and how well they feel the therapist understands them. John Gottman (Gottman, Driver, & Tabares, 2002), a psychologist who has conducted research on marriage, found he could predict divorce by studying only a few minutes of a couple's interaction with each other.

The importance of common factors in therapeutic success or failure is underscored by the fact that psychotherapies can be used with almost any patient. Put another way, only a few therapies are specific to any mental disorder. We have some evidence for specificity in relation to disorders that do not consistently respond to standard methods, particularly panic disorder and obsessive-compulsive disorder. However, most of the patients seen in primary care (and by psychiatrists) tend to have "generic" problems (particularly anxiety and mood disorders), and by and large, these patients benefit from a variety of therapeutic methods.

The Length of Therapy

Psychoanalysts believed that therapy had to be long to be effective. Freud had originally devised a treatment lasting for a few months, but by the end of his life he described psychoanalysis as intrinsically "interminable" (Freud, 1964). That in turn made for a very expensive and time-consuming procedure that few people today can afford to undergo. Indeed, as Janet Malcolm (1982) described in her book *The Impossible Profession,* even by the 1980s, very few analysts could fill a practice with analysis alone.

Although formal analysis on the couch has become a rarity, however, many therapists do still offer "psychoanalytically oriented" psychotherapy. They see patients (now seated in an armchair) once or twice a week, usually over several years. As the *Consumer Reports* survey suggested, some people appreciate this kind of therapy. And yet there is no scientific evidence supporting the effectiveness of treatment lasting for more than a year. However well intentioned those offering long-term psychotherapy may be, it is not an evidence-based practice.

Research has shown that half of all patients in therapy show no symptoms within 10 weeks, and that two thirds improve by 20 weeks (Howard, Kopta, Krause, & Orlinsky, 1986). And there is little evidence that people who fail to benefit from six months of therapy do better by continuing beyond that. Of course, one cannot say that they never do. An ideal way to test the effectiveness of longer therapy would be to assign patients to therapies of different durations. But no one has yet conducted such a study. All we can say at this point is that keeping patients in therapy for more than a few months is not justified by scientific research.

Briefer treatments have become standard, and might now be considered the "default condition" for psychotherapy. Longer term therapies are offered less often and are available only to those willing to pay out of pocket. (Insurance coverage is variable, and some policies cover only about 6 sessions a year—even though, based on the scientific data, they should allow at least 20.) The situation is rather depressing for psychiatrists and other mental health providers who may be committed to models of long-term therapy. But for those who are willing to practice on the basis of the published research, treating patients in six months makes good sense.

Even though open-ended psychotherapy with no time limit is *not* an evidence-based treatment, patients who can afford it sometimes see psychiatrists for long periods of time. The "Woody Allen model" of therapy is not just a joke. Life-long treatment exists, and we often hear about it from patients. Why do people seek long-term therapy if no evidence exists to support its effectiveness? One reason is that even when symptoms are resolved, patients still want a better quality of life. Another reason is that people always have something to talk about, and therapy gives them someone who will listen. People may also spend years searching for a magic bullet (such as discovering a childhood trauma) that they believe will resolve all their troubles. And, finally, patients and therapists who work together get attached to each other. One of my teachers told me that a therapy he was carrying out would end only when either he or the patient died (as it turned out, the therapist was the first to go). Traditional psychoanalysis, on the average, takes five to six years (Doidge et al., 2002a). However, a number of methods have been developed that prescribe a course of psychoanalytic therapy that lasts for 10–20 sessions and applies a specific focus to the patient's difficulties (Crits-Christoph & Barber, 1991). Brief dynamic therapy is the one form of psychoanalysis (if one can call it that) that has been tested over several decades—and proven effective. If Freud's model of psychoanalysis is to survive, it will probably have to be linked with such briefer modes of treatment.

Cognitive-behavioral therapy was initially designed to be relatively brief (a few months), but Beck later extended it (to last a year or two) for chronic conditions such as personality disorders (Beck, 1986). Interestingly, I have met some patients who have spent many years in CBT—for much the same reasons that others remain in psychoanalysis.

Freud was the first person to realize that therapy could become interminable, but what he did not understand is that interminability results from setting goals for treatment that are impossible to reach. If you want to be symptom-free or "completely analyzed," you are chasing an illusion. Life has many surprises for all of us, and no one lives free of psychological problems. For this reason, briefer forms of therapy make sense. But they must focus on limited goals and leave the door open for further work at a later point. When we go to a physician, even if our symptoms disappear, we do not expect that we will never need to go again. Similarly, psychotherapy can be seen as an intermittent procedure that could be useful for people at different stages of life, whenever circumstances prove too much for them. Instead of keeping patients in treatment, psychiatrists can ask their patients to try things on their own for a while and return for another course later, if necessary.

This "intermittent" model of therapy was first described by two psychoanalysts, Franz Alexander and Thomas French, as far back as 1946. It is likely that therapy is often practiced in this way, but few researchers have given intermittent therapy much attention (or studied its effectiveness).

Intermittent treatment has the advantage of countering the tendency of long-term therapies to create unnecessary dependency. (This is another point about which Alexander and French were decades ahead of their time.) Cognitive behavioral therapy and brief dynamic therapy, which can be completed in a few months, avoid the complications associated with dependency.

The problem is that if patients do not get better, therapists are reluctant to discharge them, and patients themselves may resist discharge if they do not feel better after short-term treatment. But a patient's failure to respond to treatment in the short term tends to be associated with failure to respond in the long term. For these types of refractory cases, effective treatment—be it through psychotherapy or through medication, for that matter—remains difficult to achieve.

Psychotherapy and Models of Mental Illness

All psychotherapies are based on theories about the causes of mental disorders. Psychoanalytic therapy, for example, is based on a model of inner conflict resulting from a problematic childhood. Cognitive therapy is based on a model of abnormal thoughts and emotions. These and other therapeutic theories affect the way therapy is practiced and how long it lasts.

Psychoanalysts have believed that long-term psychotherapy was necessary to counter the effects of childhood experiences. A patient's present difficulties were seen as reflections or re-creations of that patient's past. Many other "schools" of therapy took up this idea as well, and quite a few educated people still believe that experiences in childhood are the primary determinant of adult functioning. Intuitively, it seems that the way our parents raise us should shape the kind of people we become and would determine whether we develop mental disorders.

But are these assumptions really true? Do most psychological problems derive from an unhappy childhood? Many patients do describe significant problems in early life. But then so do most people—in or out of treatment. Although research shows *some* correlation between childhood adversity and adult symptoms, the link is weaker than most people believe (Rutter, 1987; Rutter & Rutter, 1993). Most children who experience an unhappy childhood (even including physical and sexual abuse) overcome these experiences and become normal adults. That is called *resilience* to adversity. We have evolved to overcome bad experiences—not to suffer endlessly. Some people are more vulnerable than others. But most are sufficiently resilient to survive adversity. Even people with a predisposition to develop symptoms may never cross the line to develop mental disorders if they are protected by a reasonable upbringing and other factors. Thus, research runs contrary to the perceived relationship between childhood and mental illness. Psychological theories along these lines have been either too simple or simply incorrect.

Why did therapists believing in such theories get this wrong? One major reason is that therapists see patients who tell impressive stories of past misery, and the therapists mistakenly infer a cause-and-effect relationship between those hardships and current symptoms. Therapists do not treat everyone who has experienced adverse events. They tend to see only people who have developed symptoms after such events. Those who have bounced back (i.e., are resilient) are in the majority but do not present to mental health professionals (Rutter, 1987; Rutter & Rutter, 1993). Thus, clinicians see only one side of the coin and often conclude that adverse life events caused their patients' psychological problems, when an event is only one of many risk factors.

Researchers have sometimes made the same mistakes, by asking psychiatric patients about their early experiences, using questionnaires or interviews specifically designed for that purpose. But the problem with this type of research is *recall bias*, where people tend to remember the past in a negative light when they are unhappy and in a more positive light when they are happier (McNally, 2003; Schachter, 1996). For this reason, we cannot simply trust recollections of the past, particularly when adults with mental disorders are asked to remember events that occurred decades ago.

The ideal way to get around this difficulty is to conduct *prospective* research. In this method, researchers directly assess life experiences in children and then follow these children into adulthood. The prospective method avoids the problem of an experience's being distorted by memory. This kind of research is usually conducted in normal community populations rather than among patients. Although it is also possible to confirm retrospective data with documents, prospective designs are generally more informative.

This research has yielded more evidence for the importance of adverse life events in adult life than for the effects of childhood experience. In an influential study led by Avshalom Caspi (a research psychologist working in Wisconsin and London), a large group of New Zealand children have been followed from birth into young adulthood. In two widely quoted papers, Caspi's group found that although genetic markers were associated with criminal behavior and depression, these outcomes occurred *only* when current life circumstances were stressful (Caspi et al., 2002, 2003).

Unfortunately, prospective research is very expensive, and we still have only a few studies that have followed large groups of children into adulthood. Still another problem is that prospective cohorts are not fully representative of the population because children from more-disturbed families are less likely to enter research studies in the first place and because they are less stable and more likely to drop out during follow-up.

Nonetheless, research consistently shows that there is no simple relationship between a bad childhood and mental illness. People who have *both* biological vulnerabilities *and* adverse life experiences are the most likely to develop problems. It takes more than bad genes or bad luck to produce mental illness.

A more fundamental problem is that continuities between childhood and adulthood may have little to do with life experience. They may simply track biological vulnerabilities that are present at all stages of development. Moreover, troubled children tend to *create* a bad environment because their problematic behavior creates difficulties for parents, teachers, and peers (Scarr & McCartney, 1983).

One way to sort out these complexities is to use *behavioral genetics* (Plomin, DeFries, McClearn, & Rutter, 2001). This method separates the effects of genes and environment, usually by comparing identical and fraternal twins. When identical twins are more similar on any trait than are fraternal twins, one can calculate the percentage of variance accounted for by genes. Behavioral genetic research has consistently shown that intelligence and personality are highly heritable and are not just the result of upbringing. These studies have also shown that almost every disorder known to psychiatry has a heritable component close to 50%.

Ironically, another challenge to the idea that childhood experience determines adult functioning comes from the other half of the equation—the relation of the environment to traits and symptoms. The behavioral genetic method can determine whether, above and beyond heredity, being brought up similarly (e.g., by the same parents) makes people more similar to each other. The data have shown, to the surprise of many, that siblings are hardly more similar than perfect strangers are. Growing up in the same family does not make people alike (Harris, 1998).

If early experiences do not produce mental illness, psychotherapy need not be based on a detailed analysis of childhood. Adverse experiences, even when associated with symptoms, do not actually *cause* disorders. Instead, *current* life experiences trigger psychological symptoms in people who are vulnerable to adverse events.

It follows that therapists should spend more time on the present and less on the past. Moreover, it has never been shown that exploring childhood is either necessary or useful. Therapies (such as cognitive-behavioral therapy) that spend little or no time on the past have more evidence for their effectiveness than do therapies (such as psychoanalysis) that spend years reviewing childhood events (Goode, 2000).

There are other reasons to question the value of psychotherapies that focus on childhood. Research has not supported the concept that adverse events produce conflicts in the mind, or that conflicts cause symptoms. Nor has research shown that exploring the unconscious mind is a necessary part of psychotherapy (Harris, 1998). Although a good part of the content of the human mind is unconscious, that does not prove that therapists must discover hidden conflicts or memories. As a colleague of mine remarked archly after 10 years of psychoanalysis, "I am still waiting for that one big insight about what happened in my childhood." Actually, that kind of drama occurs only in Hollywood movies. In real life, therapists and patients spend most of their time working on current issues. In the past, therapy focusing on the present was devalued by analysts as lacking "depth." As Aaron Beck ironically remarked, "There is more to the surface than meets the eye."

Theories that underlie psychotherapy need to be consistent with modern research showing that mental disorders occur in temperamentally susceptible people who are exposed to adverse life events. Treatment may require teaching patients to work their way around vulnerabilities. In fact, psychotherapy can be conducted without making *any* assumptions concerning the nature of mental disorders. Even when the causes of illness are almost entirely biological, psychotherapists can help patients function better.

Conclusion

Psychotherapy is one of the most effective methods of treating psychological symptoms. It does not need to be lengthy—in fact, there is good evidence that a few months' treatment is sufficient for most patients. Moreover, psychotherapy does as well as drugs for the "garden-variety" symptoms that most patients exhibit. Finally, psychotherapy saves the health care system money because patients receiving this form of treatment are less likely to ask for multiple consultations (Borus & Olendzki, 1985; Gabbard, Lazar, Hornberger, & Speigel, 1997; Paris, 2000a).

Given this strong evidence base, it is rather surprising that psychiatrists are not always trained to do psychotherapy and that they do not consistently provide (or prescribe) this form of treatment (Wilk, West, Rae, & Regier, 2006). I will examine the reasons for this paradox in Chapter 9.

PART II

DIAGNOSIS

3

Diagnosis in Psychiatry

Physicians have always treated disease by organizing signs and symptoms into diagnoses. These categories of illness are used to guide treatment. Ideally, medicine aims to prescribe specific therapies for specific diagnoses.

Thus, diagnosis is an essential skill for every physician. It provides a way for doctors to communicate with each other about illnesses and to ensure that they are discussing more or less the same thing. Because medicine is an applied science, and science always begins with what one can observe, diagnosis is a useful tool for conducting research on and developing theories about disorders. It also helps bring order to the chaos of symptoms by classifying disorders. Moreover, diagnosis provides patients with an explanation of their suffering. When treatment is known to be effective, receiving a diagnosis can provide relief and hope.

Medical diagnosis has evolved over the last century, even though the causes of many diseases remain unknown. In the past, physicians classified diseases on the basis of clinical observations. Today diagnosis has come to depend on an understanding of pathological mechanisms.

Ultimately, categorization has to be rooted in both the *causes* of disease (etiology) and in the *process* of disease (pathogenesis).

For example, cerebral thrombosis, one of the main types of stroke, has a specific pathogenesis (a clot blocks an artery leading to the brain). However, researchers are still working on the etiology of stroke, that is, why clots form in the first place.

When diseases were classified on the basis of symptoms alone, medicine recognized only a few categories. Today, scientific research allows us to identify an increasing number of diseases. The more precise medical knowledge becomes, the more likely it will be that treatment follows logically from diagnosis.

Psychiatric Diagnosis

The concept of psychiatric diagnosis is an especially thorny one these days—and, in fact, in no other field of medicine are there as many endless controversies about diagnosis as there are in psychiatry. Why? Because, first and foremost, psychiatrists lack sufficient understanding of the etiology or pathogenesis of mental disorders; therefore, diagnostic parameters in psychiatry cannot be defined as well as those in other domains of medicine can be. Moreover, some critics of psychiatry dismiss the diagnostic process in psychiatry as nothing more than the "labeling" of human problems, or else say that it is dehumanizing (Scheff, 1966). For severe mental disorders, such as schizophrenia, bipolar illness, and melancholic depression, such criticism is misguided and naïve. These conditions are little different in their degree of harm to patients than are the serious diseases that other physicians treat.

On the other hand, critiques of psychiatric diagnosis have greater relevance for patients with less severe symptoms that may be a normal, albeit painful, variation of human emotions or cognitive experiences. The current diagnostic system of psychiatry fails to recognize these variations and to distinguish between pathology and normality. And critics are not entirely wrong in seeing a dark side to such categorization. Psychiatrists can easily lose sight of the person suffering a given set of symptoms when they become too concerned about finding the "correct" diagnosis of a supposed disease. They tend to forget that patients do not have only symptoms but strengths as well—positive coping mechanisms that can help them recover from illness and live meaningful lives.

The problem for psychiatry is not with the concept of diagnosis itself but with *invalid* diagnosis. Diagnoses are an essential part of psychiatry. They are a practical way to organize symptoms and, when valid, often provide useful guidelines to treatment. But unlike well-defined diagnoses in other fields of medicine, only a few psychiatric diagnoses have been fully validated; the rest are makeshifts in the absence of something better. Ideally, every specific diagnosis should correspond to a unique disease process. But again, we do not yet understand the mechanisms behind mental illness. It is this significant gap in our knowledge that renders most psychiatric diagnoses provisional rather than "real." Most research that is based on these provisional assumptions (e.g., epidemiological research on the prevalence of major depressive disorder) consequently relies on uncertain terms. Treatment decisions often rest on equally shaky grounds.

Biological Markers and the Challenge for Psychiatric Diagnosis

A hundred years ago, medical diagnosis depended almost entirely on accurate observation. Patients were asked to describe their complaints in detail, after which physicians placed stethoscopes on chests and listened for the sounds of air passing though the lungs or of heart valves opening and closing. When I went to medical school, these procedures still had a certain mystique, and we all had to learn them. Yet diagnosis had already been made more accurate by the use of X-rays. In later years radioactive tracers allowed us to accurately visualize every organ in the body. In recent years practicing physicians sometimes hardly ever take their stethoscopes out of their pockets.

The laboratory has made physical examination less central to medicine. By the end of the 19th century it was possible to diagnose infectious diseases by culturing organisms in a laboratory. When physicians learned to use blood tests that measure body chemistry, the accuracy of diagnosis greatly increased.

Sometimes blood work does not tell you anything you do not already know. Yet it often provides a precision that physical examination alone cannot. It is one thing to feel the size and shape of a patient's liver. It is quite another to measure liver function with a battery of blood tests. There is really no substitute for some of the laboratory tests physicians perform: taking measurements of thyroid hormones, or of sodium and potassium levels. With automation, you can conduct a large number of tests at minimal expense. The same is true of scanning: It may not be necessary to listen to a patient's chest if you can look at a detailed picture of the heart and lungs.

Medical specialists have a tendency to overrate the value of blood tests and scans, and probably order too many of them. Yet there can be no doubt that biological markers have greatly advanced scientific medicine. Psychiatrists, like other physicians, need to anchor their observations in biological markers that are reliable and independent of personal bias. Such measurements provide a solid ground to diagnosis that cannot be obtained from signs and symptoms alone. That is what psychiatry lacks and what it so badly needs.

Thus, in the absence of biological markers for disease that could establish clear boundaries between one illness and another, and between illness and normality, diagnosis of mental disorders is, to say the least, difficult. The conditions we treat may be brain diseases, but we cannot biopsy a brain. Even if we could, we probably would not know what to look for. Our current understanding of the brain is simply too primitive, in comparison to what is known about the liver, the kidney, or the heart. The diseases that neurologists treat can usually be located somewhere in the brain. But in most mental disorders, the brain looks relatively normal. When physical changes in the brain do occur, they tend to be subtle. We cannot say that schizophrenia arises from one part of the brain and depression from another.

Most of the disorders psychiatrists treat have unknown causes, and the mechanisms by which symptoms develop are likewise unknown. Thus we lack the basis for accurate diagnosis that other specialties have. Most of the categories we use are *not* diseases in the same sense that breast cancer or coronary artery disease are diseases.

Medicine traditionally distinguishes among symptoms, syndromes, and diseases. *Symptoms* are subjective complaints (as opposed to *signs,* which are observable). *Syndromes* are collections of signs and symptoms that occur together but may or may not arise from a common cause or a common mechanism. As currently defined, most mental disorders are syndromes. That is why psychiatry's official classification fudges the problem by describing its categories as *disorders* rather than diseases.

The *Diagnostic and Statistical Manual of Mental Disorders* (DSM) is the standard manual of diagnosis for mental health professionals in North America and many other parts of the world; the current edition is the DSM-IV-TR (American Psychiatric Association, 2000).[1] (The World Health Organization has its own manual, the *International Classification of Diseases*, now in its 10th edition [ICD-10]; although the latter is standard in Europe and Asia, it is rarely used in North America. For a complete discussion of these issues, see Sadler [2004].) Almost all psychiatrists have a copy of the DSM in their offices. The system is popular and useful. It ensures that psychiatrists can communicate effectively about the patients they see. However, because the classification of mental disorders in the manual is provisional and pragmatic only, many (if not most) of its categories are problematic—based on "criteria," or collections of signs and symptoms describing how patients behave and what they tell us. As long as that remains the case, most psychiatric diagnoses will lack validity and fail to be an accurate guide to treatment.

This validity problem has not prevented some psychiatrists from acting as if their diagnoses describe an ultimate truth. Given the rampant practice of offering drugs to almost all patients, some clinicians favor diagnostic categories that lead to familiar prescriptions. Thus, patients who meet criteria for major depression will be prescribed an antidepressant. Patients who meet criteria for an anxiety disorder may also receive an antidepressant. Patients who have a diagnosis for which there is no specific drug can be fitted into one that leads to the prescription of an antidepressant.

The main motivation behind current practice is that psychiatrists do not want to be isolated from medicine. They want to be like other physicians. This helps explain why the profession has taken up diagnosis so enthusiastically. We want to believe we can diagnose patients accurately and prescribe treatment specific to these categories. However, with our present knowledge, these beliefs are unjustified. Although diagnosis is a necessary tool for psychiatry, the categories we use are not as real as those of stroke or tuberculosis. We may be able to establish scientifically valid diagnoses in the future, but our current knowledge is insufficient to allow us to do so.

How the DSM System Addressed Problems of Diagnosis

The problems of psychiatric diagnosis used to be even worse than they are now. Thirty or forty years ago, researchers found that practitioners could not agree about how to classify the most common types of mental illness. This fact was sometimes used to question the validity of *any* diagnosis in psychiatry.

In 1952 the American Psychiatric Association (APA) published the first edition of the DSM, followed by the DSM-II in 1968.[1] Few psychiatrists took either edition seriously: Their criteria for diagnosis had never been systematically researched, and many of their descriptions were so vague that clinicians, when referring to the book, could not even agree on whether a patient did or did not have one symptom or another. Moreover, because there were no specific treatments for specific disorders, psychiatrists often felt that splitting hairs about diagnosis was useless. (Patients with psychosis all got the same medication, and psychotherapy was not specific to any category.)

The situation changed in the 1960s, when classification began to matter. Psychiatrists now had effective drugs to be applied with some degree of specificity: Antipsychotics worked best against psychosis, whereas antidepressants worked best against depression. The introduction of lithium as a treatment for bipolar disorder meant that, depending on diagnosis, psychotic patients needed to be prescribed other drugs.

By the 1970s some academic psychiatrists began to suggest that illnesses in psychiatry were no different from those in medicine and that diagnoses should be validated through biological processes (Robins & Guze, 1970). Research showed that classification could be made reliable by using observable criteria and by following procedural rules (algorithms). The endless confusion about diagnosis could not continue, lest psychiatry lose all credibility.

In response to the growing demand for diagnostic reliability, the American Psychiatric Association sponsored the development of a new and revised DSM system. This was a major turning point in the field—a paradigm shift that changed everything. The APA put Robert Spitzer, a psychiatrist and a professor at Columbia University, in charge of this effort. The manual he developed, the DSM-III, was published in 1980 and became a best-seller, with worldwide influence. Its central principle was *reliability*, given the premise that diagnoses cannot be valid (i.e., measure what they are supposed to measure) until they are first reliable (i.e., produce consistent results).

The DSM-III largely ended arguments between psychiatrists by ending the use of idiosyncratic criteria to make diagnoses. To maximize reliability, every DSM category—and this is true of the more recent edition, the DSM-IV-TR, as well—requires the clinician to assess a set of specific criteria and then to follow a sequence to establish a diagnosis. If the manual is used correctly, most people should reach the same conclusion (subject to inevitable judgment calls). Assuming that everyone is trained to identify symptoms in the same way, one need only count. The DSM asks the clinician to determine whether a patient has a sufficient number of criteria (e.g., 5 out of 9 for major depression) to make a diagnosis. This has sometimes been called a "Chinese menu" approach. The problem is that, although reliability is needed to produce validity, reliability does not necessarily prove anything about validity. We can all agree and all still be wrong.

Another crucial element of the DSM-III is that it defined mental disorders entirely on the basis of clinical symptoms and course, rather than on theories about the causes of illness. In most ways the "atheoretical" approach of the DSM-III was a great advance. Deriving diagnoses from unproven theories had been one of the main problems with the DSM-I and DSM-II. (For example, both editions asked psychiatrists to diagnose what were then called neuroses on the basis of "unconscious conflicts.") The DSM-III focused on symptoms, recognizing that psychiatrists have insufficient data to explain the mechanisms behind most mental disorders.

But the DSM-III had its conceptual problems as well: Because valid diagnoses are based on the causes, not the symptoms, of illness, the DSM categories are little more than useful abstractions. The DSM remains an incomplete blueprint for identifying, researching, and guiding treatment for most mental disorders. The absence of knowledge—still decades away, as noted previously—about the underlying causes of mental disorders leaves the field, and the DSM, essentially no choice but to identify these disorders based on patient-reported symptoms and clinician-observed signs, all of which are subjective (i.e., vulnerable to bias and faulty judgment) and definitional moving targets in the absence of well-understood etiology and pathogenesis. Nevertheless, many practitioners do not understand the limitations of the DSM, particularly the reality that most of its categories are syndromes. Nor is it always clear how mental disorder, as defined by the DSM, differs from normality.

The problem with basing diagnosis on observable features is that different diseases produce similar symptoms. That is how medicine made diagnoses in the past. For example, inflammation, anemia, jaundice, and paralysis were all treated as diseases. Of course, these terms describe only symptoms or syndromes that reflect a wide variety of underlying processes and pathologies.

Nonetheless, there is a point that occasionally has gotten lost in the various debates about the DSM in recent years: Considering how little is known about mental illnesses, psychiatrists still do a reasonable job of managing patients, and most provide as good service as do other medical specialists. It is certainly possible to help people in distress without understanding precisely why they get sick. But to do better, psychiatrists need to gain greater knowledge through etiological research. Until that happens, the DSM system provides a common language by which psychiatrists and other mental health professionals can communicate with each other. That alone represents a significant step in the field.

The Reification of Diagnosis

The past few decades have provided an opportunity to study the categories listed in the DSM-III; but with a few minor exceptions, the system has remained the same. Over the years, people forgot that the process that created each edition of the manual was not based strictly on scientific evidence but on expert consensus. In time, a *reification* of the DSM has occurred. Indeed, a generation has passed since the DSM-III was introduced, and diagnosis has taken on a reality of its own—one that it does not deserve. In the research world, one can no longer publish a scientific paper on mental illness without applying DSM categories to subjects. Doing so offers a degree of confidence that the findings can be replicated in other populations. On the other hand, patients meeting criteria for any DSM diagnosis are often heterogeneous (i.e., significantly different from one another). Thus, placing a group of patients in a category, however reliably, gives the false impression that a particular group of symptoms corresponds to a unique form of disease.

In the clinical world, practitioners tend to assume that a diagnosis explains what is wrong with a patient. That is rarely the case in psychiatry.

DSM categories obscure important individual differences in etiology and pathogenesis. Patients falling into a category are often too heterogeneous to predict treatment response: having the same diagnosis does not necessarily predict that people will respond in the same way. (Chapter 5 will describe how different from one another are people diagnosed with major depression.)

Another problem is that the DSM encourages psychiatrists to give patients multiple diagnoses (First, 2005). We often speak of *comorbidity*, that is, the overlap between disorders—as if two *separate* diseases existed in the same patient. But comorbidity is an illusion because DSM categories are syndromes, not medical diseases. For example, one of the most common comorbidities, that between substance abuse and depression, obscures the fact that people may drink or take drugs because of low mood and that the consequences of doing so can make them even more depressed. Another common example, the comorbidity of depression and anxiety (the most common psychiatric presentation in medical practice) obscures the likelihood that both derive from a single process (Goldberg & Goodyer, 2005).

Another problem with diagnoses of mental illness is how to weigh the vulnerability factors that underlie disorders. Life circumstances form part of the context of mental disorders. Another part of the context derives from any personality traits of the patient that will make it more (or less) likely that symptoms will develop. Still another contributing factor is the patient's overall functional level (often more clinically relevant than the diagnosis itself).

This is why the DSM introduced its five-axis system of coding. Symptomatic disorders are coded on Axis I. Personality traits and personality disorders are coded on Axis II. Medical illnesses are coded on Axis III. Axis IV codes are for life stressors. Axis V scores the patient's functional level.

However, most practitioners do not have the time for this level of complexity. Like other physicians, they are interested in symptoms they can treat. In my experience, many psychiatrists diagnose patients on Axis I only and leave the rest to researchers. In any case, the zeitgeist encourages us to believe that the only "real" pathology lies in symptoms, as opposed to behavioral patterns over time.

In summary, the reification of the DSM reflects the slow progress of research on the causes and processes behind mental illness. There are many unsolved problems with the validity of categories in the DSM system. Is schizophrenia one illness or many? Is major depression one illness, or are different types of depression separate diseases? These questions have not been answered. Yet in the absence of something better, the categories created by the DSM-III have taken on a life of their own. The DSM-IV, when published in 1994, was explicitly designed to provide stability and established those categories even more firmly. The text revision of the DSM-IV, published in 2000, was simply an expansion of the 1994 text, with few changes in its diagnostic criteria. The DSM-V should be released in 2012, but it is unlikely to introduce radical changes. There is a good reason for that. The expansion of knowledge in psychiatry—again, especially in the area of disease causes and process—has not been sufficient for a major revision or for any sort of paradigm change of the magnitude represented by the DSM-III. Thus, the essential concepts introduced in 1980 will likely remain in place.

All the same, the DSM-V revision could be a great opportunity for the field. The process is in the hands of David Kupfer, the chair of the psychiatry department at the University of Pittsburgh (one of the world's great centers for psychiatric research), and Darryl Regier, a psychiatric epidemiologist who has worked for many years for the American Psychiatric Association. In 2004 Regier told me that the APA wants to be sure that the next version will be more strongly based in data—and that this time they want to take the time "to get it right." One can only hope they succeed.

In 2002 Kupfer and Regier (along with Michael First, a professor at Columbia) published a book entitled *A Research Agenda for DSM-V* (Kupfer, First, & Regier, 2002). Hearteningly, the authors were clearly aware of the most important issues in the process of preparing the new manual. These include the overall definition of a mental disorder, and the need for diagnostic criteria based on etiology and pathogenesis and a place for the role of culture in shaping symptoms.

If the DSM-V truly follows a research agenda, it could be a great improvement over its predecessors. However, it still has to cope with limited empirical data. The danger is that political considerations within the field will fill the gap and that the final product will reflect more about clinical psychiatrists' interest in justifying what they do than about medical science.

Inventing New Diagnoses

The pitfalls of writing a diagnostic manual are well illustrated by some of the suggestions that have been made for new categories that might be added to the DSM-V. Most have to do with validating activities that psychiatrists perform that are not strictly related to mental disorders.

For example, psychiatrists and psychologists who do family therapy may have no diagnostic code to use for insurance purposes. They have therefore suggested that we add a new category of *relational disorders,* defined as dysfunctions in relationships between people (Kupfer et al., 2002). This concept could also be used to describe the problems that many patients bring to individual psychotherapy. But if you are in treatment because you cannot get along with your spouse, do you have a mental disorder at all? We should also ask whether psychiatrists should actually spend their time treating relational disorders. Defining all psychological problems as disorders can become a political and social act that does not correspond to what physicians have always considered medical diagnoses.

The fact is that anyone can come up with a list of criteria written in "DSMese" that will be no better and no worse than the ones we have been living with since 1980. However, adding more diagnostic categories to the present mess is no solution. Instead, we should limit the scope of the DSM to diagnoses of conditions that are unquestionably mental disorders, and ensure that any additions have good research behind them.

Structured Interviews

A related problem for the DSM system concerns attempts to make current categories more scientific by using standardized interviews that produce reliable results. In the past, psychiatrists had idiosyncratic methods of making diagnoses. The DSM system was designed to prevent that from happening. When you use a standard list of criteria, everyone has to ask the same questions and understand the answers to those questions in the same way.

Structured interviews were developed to make this process even more reliable. Interviewers were instructed to use written questions, and raters were trained to turn answers into standardized scores. A large body of such instruments have been developed, many of which are based directly on DSM criteria. The most widely used instrument, the Structured Interview for Mental Disorders, Axis I (SCID-I), essentially reproduces the DSM criteria while priming the interviewer to ensure that all relevant questions are asked, and the SCID-II does the same for personality disorders (First, Spitzer, Gibbon, & Williams, 1997a, 1997b). When everyone is reading the same playbook, diagnoses are indeed more reliable. The problem is, again, that an invalid diagnosis, or a diagnosis with unclear boundaries, can also be reliable, even if supported by a structured interview. If the gold standard derives from DSM criteria, then instruments developed to diagnose a specific disorder will be no better than the DSM itself. In short, structured interviews, however useful they may be for clinical research, give clinical diagnosis an undeserved scientific gloss. They improve reliability but do nothing to solve the problem of validity.

Consider the following example. Marlene Steinberg, a Yale psychiatrist interested in multiple personality disorder, developed a diagnostic interview called the Structured Clinical Interview for DSM-IV Dissociative Disorders-Revised (SCID-D). (She obtained permission from Spitzer to use the SCID acronym, which provided this measure with a degree of credibility.) However, there is doubt as to whether there is any such thing as multiple personality disorder (see Chapter 5). Thus, the nonexistence of a disease in no way prevents people from diagnosing it with an instrument that purports to be scientific.

The Prevalence Game

Physicians passionately interested in any disease tend to believe it is receiving insufficient attention, especially in terms of funding. Obtaining funds for treatment and research is greatly influenced by the prevalence of a disorder in the general population. Thus, the greater the number of people with a particular psychiatric diagnosis, the more money we need to spend to identify and treat that particular disorder. As a researcher, I know that the first sentence of every grant application must focus on the prevalence of the disorder under study.

To determine the rate of mental disorders in the community, researchers conduct large-scale epidemiological surveys. The first of these, made in the 1980s, was the Epidemiological Catchment Area (ECA) Study, a door-to-door survey in five areas of the United States, supported by the National Institute for Mental Health (NIMH) (Robins & Regier, 1991). A decade later, a second study, the National Comorbidity Survey (NCS) was conducted (Kessler et al., 1994). More recently, an even more sophisticated project, the National Comorbidity Survey Replication (NCS-R), has been carried out (Kessler, Chiu, Demler, Merikangas, & Walters, 2005).

These surveys have provided data about the prevalence of DSM-defined mental disorders in the American population. The main results of the NCS-R were published in June 2005 in the *Archives of General Psychiatry* by a team led by Ronald Kessler of Harvard (Kessler et al., 2005). One of the study's most striking findings was that nearly half of the population met criteria for at least one DSM disorder in their lifetime and that 26% suffer from a mental disorder in any given year.

Depending on one's point of view, one might react to these figures with incredulity or indifference. Are the results exaggerated or factual? All the numbers depend on the validity of DSM categories. Inevitably, all the difficulties associated with the DSM system afflict epidemiological research.

The New York Times published a series of articles on the NCS-R report (Carey, 2005a, 2005b). Kessler was asked whether mental disorders are defined in a way that makes them highly prevalent. Kessler replied that no one is surprised at the much higher (and universal) prevalence of physical illness. If half of the population has a medical condition in the course of a year (and if all have physical illness in the course of a lifetime), then why should the prevalence of mental disorders be any different? In Kessler's view, the findings are controversial only because of the enduring stigma associated with mental illness. But the reporter still wanted to know whether mental disorder loses meaning when used to describe symptoms experienced by most people. If half of us meet criteria for a mental disorder, does the concept distinguish pathology from normality?

In an *Archives* editorial that accompanied a series of articles from NCS-R data, two psychiatrists from the National Institute of Mental Health, Thomas Insel and Wayne Fenton, asked: "What should we make of these numbers? If one quarter of the population has a disorder each year, are most mental disorders so mild as to be trivial? Or are these disorders serious and more prevalent but under-reported?" (Insel & Fenton, 2005, p. 590).

The NCS-R also found that many more people have disorders than are in treatment. This result seems to suggest that mental illness remains unrecognized and untreated. If so, psychiatry might need more priority within the medical field. But which disorders are being untreated? If schizophrenia, bipolar disorder, and melancholia are the ones being missed, then patients are indeed missing out on effective treatment for serious illnesses. But if people with mild depressions are not coming for help, we could be less concerned.

A related question concerns whether the DSM should include mild or "subclinical" disorders in its classification. The concept of *diagnostic spectra* suggests that there may be no absolute separation between milder and more severe disorders. Again, Kessler, who favors inclusiveness, points out that the rest of medicine has never excluded subclinical conditions from its classification system (Kessler et al., 2003).

Nonetheless, the overall high prevalence of disorders in the NCS-R is based on a very broad definition of mental illness. Most cases fall into a few, common categories (Kessler et al., 2005). Alcohol abuse has a lifetime prevalence of 13%, and social phobia has a prevalence of 12%, whereas major depression can affect more than 16% of people over a lifetime. But because all of these conditions have fuzzy boundaries, they may have been overestimated by the use of DSM criteria for diagnosis.

We also cannot assume that these population estimates are any more valid than DSM itself. There are also problems of measurement. The frequency of simple phobias is an example. The community prevalence of these conditions (fear attached to highly specific situations or things) was examined by the ECA study, which was conducted in several American cities and one rural area. By and large, major mental disorders had similar prevalence rates at each site (about 6%), but there was an anomaly in that Baltimore had a rate of 11% (Robins & Regier, 1991).

There was no reason to think that Baltimore was an unusually frightening place. The problem was that because there is no absolute boundary between normal fears and diagnosable phobias, scoring at one site can easily become aberrant. The research assistants were probably using too low a threshold. Many phobic symptoms have no clinical significance. (It has sometimes been said that the best results for the efficacy of behavior therapy were obtained by treating snake phobias in urban dwellers.) The same problem emerged in the NCS-R study, which found a lifetime prevalence of 12% for simple phobia.

The systematic diagnostic criteria in the DSM scheme provide researchers with a tool to ascertain the prevalence of mental disorders in the community. But we see the same problem as in structured interviews. We are measuring prevalence using DSM categories that may or may not be valid. The gold standard turns out to be made of copper.

The prevalence problem is important because it can determine who wins and who loses. The greater the number of people with mental disorders, the more money flowing toward psychiatry. The greater the number of people with any specific type of disorder, the more money flowing in that specific direction.

This is one reason that experts interested in specific disorders tend to inflate their prevalence. But over-diagnosis, generally based on theoretical biases, has a long history in psychiatry. There was a time when a generation of psychiatrists diagnosed all neurotic symptoms as "masked depression" (Razali, 2000). But whereas mood symptoms can be seen in many conditions, this does not prove they are the underlying problem. If everything in psychiatry were really depression, what meaning would be left for the concept?

More recently, bipolar disorder, formerly considered to have a prevalence of about 1%, has been claimed to affect 10% of the general population, mainly because all of its purported spectrum manifestations—depression, substance abuse, and personality disorders—have been included (see discussion in Chapter 4). Finally, the newly "discovered" diagnosis of social phobia has shot up in prevalence from less than 1% to 13%, as experts have written about it and as industry has promoted treatment for it (Wakefield, Horwitz, & Schmitz, 2005).

It sometimes seems as if any human problem can be turned into a psychiatric diagnosis. The DSM system has encouraged that trend and does not tell us how to distinguish between mental illness and life. Although serious efforts have been made to narrow the scope of mental disorder, psychiatrists need to have a concept of normality against which true illness can be described (Offer & Sabshin, 1966; Wakefield, 1992; Wakefield & First, 2003).

Diagnosis in the Courtroom

One of the more troubling aspects of the DSM system is the way it has been used in the courts. Defense lawyers who need to get their clients

acquitted are sorely tempted to offer a psychiatric diagnosis as a mitigating factor. Although this problem did not start with the DSM, the
reification of categories has made it more serious.

Criminal law has a rather narrow definition of an insanity defense
(see Chapter 12). This defense is usually limited to situations in which
criminal acts are carried out under the influence of psychotic delusions
(Robinson, 1996). However, other DSM diagnoses have crept into the
law. Very few courts would accept antisocial personality (a diagnosis very
common among prisoners) as a defense because its criteria are actually
based (in part) on a pattern of long-term criminal behavior. There have
also been cases in which defendants claimed to act when in a dissociated
state (or an alternate personality) (Halleck, 1990). There have even been
cases where premenstrual syndrome (found in the appendix of the DSM)
was invoked as a mitigating factor (Downs, 2002). Now that bipolar
illness is being used to explain all forms of irrational conduct, it is likely to
be entered as a defense in the courtroom, even for people who have never
been hospitalized or treated.

When psychiatric diagnosis takes on the entire world, lawyers can
seize on these categories to defend their clients against any criminal
charge. And if half of us meet the criteria for a DSM diagnosis at some
time in our lives, is there any room left for the concept of criminal
responsibility?

Why Diagnosis Is Not a Guide to Treatment

One of the most serious problems in clinical practice today is the way the
DSM system of diagnosis has been used as a guide to treatment. In
principle, using it thus is not a bad idea. But first we need valid diagnoses
based on disease processes. Only then can we develop treatments specific to categories. Diagnoses that have not been validated cannot be a
useful guide to treatment.

The DSM manual explicitly eschewed any link between diagnosis
and treatment. The DSM is a practical system that was never intended to
determine which treatments should be offered to patients. The problem
is that psychiatrists, trained as physicians, want to believe that the current system can do the job. That is why so many depressed patients
receive antidepressants—even when the clinical picture calls into
question their efficacy (Delate, Gelenberg, Simmons, & Motheral, 2004;

Olfson et al., 2002; Paulose-Ram, Safran, Jonas, Gu, Orwig, in press; Raymond et al., 2007).

The concept that drugs should be "indicated" for a specific condition is now deeply ingrained in medicine. In the 1960s, after the thalidomide scandal (in which an inadequately tested agent caused serious birth defects), the Food and Drug Administration established guidelines for approving new drugs, based on their efficacy for diagnostic categories. This model is definitely appropriate for infectious diseases, where research dictates that antibiotics be prescribed for one disease but not for another. It is also valid for choosing drug treatments for heart disease and cancer.

But the model does not apply well to psychiatric drugs. The agents we use are just not that specific. They resemble analgesics or anti-inflammatory agents in that they produce similar effects on symptoms in entirely different diseases.

In the older psychiatry, patients, irrespective of diagnosis, were often offered the same treatment (i.e., psychotherapy) for *every* symptom. Today, too many psychiatrists believe that mental disorders reflect disordered chemistry that can be made right by the proper combination of drugs. Although the future should bring more valid diagnoses and better therapeutic methods, the idea that current diagnoses can guide treatment is illusory.

Conclusion

Diagnosis is essential for psychiatry, but the reification of invalid categories leads to invalid clinical practices. Even the most common disorders, such as major depression, describe a heterogeneous group of problems that do not respond to a single treatment.

I do not agree with broadside attacks on the DSM system—or the paranoid view that psychiatrists want to define everyone as mentally ill in order to increase the power of their profession. (This interpretation greatly exaggerates the influence of psychiatry on society—we can only wish we were as powerful as our critics seem to think we are.) Psychiatrists need a diagnostic system in psychiatry, and the DSM, for all its faults, is the best we have come up with yet.

The problem is that the very success of the DSM system has led many psychiatrists to see the DSM as more than it really is. As a practical way of communicating information about patients in a diagnostic "shorthand," the DSM is a success. But when clinicians reify psychiatric diagnoses and use them (unjustifiably) as precise guides to treatment, practice suffers. To make matters worse, researchers keep proposing new categories. (Anyone can write a set of criteria in the style of the DSM and lobby for their inclusion in the next manual.)

Again, the great achievement of the DSM system was that it provided a common language for research and practice. While waiting for more scientific data, we should not see the system as a given but as a station on the way to deeper knowledge. I teach my students to learn the DSM thoroughly but not to consider it as *true*. The manual provides us with a system that is better than what came before it but that can and should be expected to undergo radical change over time.

It is worth considering what the DSM might look like 50 or 100 years from now. If we could identify the biological processes behind illness, the current manual might turn out to be no more valid than medical diagnoses from the 19th century. Some syndromes may turn out to be caused by single diseases. Others may split into many separate diagnostic entities. One thing is for sure: The DSM of the future will not be based on symptoms alone but will make use of biological markers—once they are discovered (First & Zimmerman, 2006).

4

The Boundaries of
Mental Disorders

M ost people experience psychological symptoms from time to time—most of us know, for example, what it feels like to be anxious or depressed. Does that mean that everyone has a mental illness? What is the boundary between mental disorder and the normal emotional experiences, the ups and downs, of everyday life?

In medicine, *illness* (or disease) describes a process leading to impairment of normal physiological function. However, we do not know enough about the brain to describe mental symptoms on the basis of physiology. For this reason, we are not really justified in using the terms "disease" or "illness" in psychiatry. As an alternative to that terminology, and in one of its major innovations, the DSM-III introduced the term "mental disorder," which is defined in the DSM-IV-TR as:

> a clinically significant behavioral or psychological syndrome or pattern that occurs in an individual and that is associated with present distress (e.g., a painful symptom) or disability (i.e., impairment in one or more important areas of functioning) with a significantly increased risk of suffering, death, personal disability,

or an important loss of freedom. In addition, this syndrome or pattern must not be merely an expectable and culturally sanctioned response to a particular event, for example, the death of a loved one. Whatever its original cause, it must currently be considered a manifestation of a behavioral, psychological, or biological dysfunction in the individual. Neither deviant behavior (e.g., political, religious, or sexual) nor conflicts that are primarily between the individual and society are mental disorders unless the deviance or conflict is a symptom of a dysfunction in the individual, as described above. (American Psychiatric Association, 2000, pp. xxi–xxii)

It is hard to know where to begin in critiquing this definition. In spite of an attempt to be scientific, much remains subjective. For example, what is meant by "clinically significant"? Who decides what is significant—the doctor, the patient, or society? What is the meaning of "dysfunction"? Virtually any psychological symptom makes you less functional than you would be if you did not have it.

Consider some specific examples. If someone is depressed after the death of a loved one, how can we know what is "expectable" and what is not? If criminals are in conflict with society, does that reflect a dysfunction in the individual or in the social environment?

In practice, using a definition without established boundaries can lead psychiatric diagnosis to take on the whole universe of human problems. Defining mental disorders so broadly simply fails to distinguish among illness, unhappiness, misbehavior, and eccentricity.

Mental disorder as a concept seems to fall on a continuum somewhere between illness and normality. Some of the most severe conditions we treat (schizophrenia, classical bipolar illness, and melancholic depression) are in fact like medical diseases. At the other end of the continuum, some of the mental disorders listed in DSM-IV-TR (e.g., phobias in adults and oppositional defiant disorder in children) are not easily separated from problems that normal people have.

Thus, despite the disclaimer in the last sentence of the definition quoted above, there is no precise way to distinguish a mental disorder from an expectable response to life stressors. The DSM system describes levels of symptoms that define disorder somewhat arbitrarily. And if one fails to meet the criteria for any Axis I condition, one may still have an "adjustment disorder" (which is not considered an illness). Moreover, the high prevalence of many disorders, as defined by the DSM system, also demonstrates a problem with boundaries.

Jerome Wakefield, a professor at New York University with a background in social work, has made a useful contribution to the problem of defining mental disorders, suggesting a narrower concept based on what he calls "harmful dysfunction" (Horwitz & Wakefield, 2007). Wakefield's term combines two principles: (1) that a disorder is harmful; and (2) that a disorder is a dysfunction (i.e., an inability of some internal mechanism to perform its natural evolutionary function). In this view, one would not have a disorder unless symptoms could be shown to meet both criteria. Nonetheless, Wakefield's proposal does not avoid the problems of asking clinicians to make judgment calls about what is harmful and about what is dysfunctional. We need to find a way to ground the concept of harmful dysfunction in objective indicators such as biological markers.

To describe what is "dysfunctional" one also needs to define *normality.* That term has been understood in various ways in psychiatry (Horwitz & Wakefield, 2007). One way is to define normal as average. But at least half of us will meet criteria for a DSM-defined mental disorder at some time in our lives. Thus, by that definition, it is normal to be sick—at least from time to time.

Another option is to define normality as an optimal state in which people have no symptoms and function well in all aspects of their lives. Of course, no such state can exist—at least not for long. DSM-IV-TR has a system (on Axis V) for scoring people, on a scale of 1 to 100, on their level of functioning. (I have never seen a patient in treatment score above 70, and I suspect that no one I know ever reaches a score of 80 for more than a week at a time—and that usually happens on vacation.)

Although entire books have been written about normality in psychiatry, we still have no objective way to define it. Normal life is full of problems. We all have periods in which work is disrupted and relationships are in danger. We all experience symptoms from time to time.

Thus, the DSM is so inclusive that the entire human condition itself lies within its pages. When we categorize all psychological problems as mental disorders, we end up with a system that tries to cover everything but explains nothing while at the same time "pathologizing" some of the very traits that make us human. In a recent book (coauthored by Allen

Horwitz), Wakefield points out that the classical concept of depression, in which severe symptoms emerge with few precipitants, has been conflated with sadness, in which symptoms develop parallel to losses and stressors (Horwitz & Wakefield, 2007). (Chapter 5 will examine this problem in some detail.)

We would have an easier time of it if the DSM diagnosed only patients with serious mental disorders. To do so, it would need to establish meaningful cutoff points that clearly separate pathology from the outer ranges of normality. However, this type of boundary would exclude many of the patients seen by mental health professionals. Because one of the functions of the DSM is to describe the conditions that psychiatrists treat (and can bill for), narrowing the definition of mental disorders would be a disaster for psychiatrists who depend on insurance.

There is also a more theoretical argument against restricting the domain of psychiatry only to patients who are severely ill. Ronald Kessler, the leader of the NCS-R study, suggests that mental illness, like physical illness, should not be expected to have sharp boundaries (Kessler et al., 2003). Similar issues arise in the rest of medicine. Do high levels of cholesterol describe a disease or merely a normal variation? Do some cancerous cells in the prostate reflect the beginning of a life-threatening disease or just a normal effect of aging? It should not be surprising that mental disorders flow into a number of milder conditions that lie in a spectrum with types that are more severe. Nonetheless, these variations related to medical diseases are all based on biological measures—not judgment calls.

Diagnosing the World

Psychiatry's wanting to include more (or most) people among those with a diagnosis of mental disorder has a number of causes. First, the DSM system fails to ground its categories in objective measures. Second, because of the nature of psychiatric practice, in which many patients have milder forms of disorder, insurance companies require a diagnosis before it will pay for treatment. Finally, the pharmaceutical industry plays a role in promoting diagnoses. Because its responsibility is to its stockholders and not to patients, the industry's priority is to increase sales of its products (its medications), and so a broadly defined array of diagnoses for which those medications can be prescribed serves the industry's ultimate agenda. There are great profits to be made in industry if everyone has a mental disorder. For example, if every shy person with a diagnosis of social anxiety disorder were on an antidepressant, the pharmaceutical industry could earn additional billions of dollars.

But in fact such treatment does not prove that a mental disorder is present. As Chapter 8 will show, the medications we use work on a wide variety of symptoms and psychological problems. In fact, drugs such as antidepressants might even improve the quality of life for *normal* people (Kramer, 1993).

Another example of psychiatry seeming to "diagnose the world" can be seen in a 2006 epidemiological paper in the *Archives of General Psychiatry* that examined the prevalence of a condition called *intermittent explosive disorder* (IED) (Kessler et al., 2006). This diagnosis is included in the DSM-IV-TR but is rarely used. IED is defined by "several discrete episodes of failure to resist aggressive impulses that result in serious assaultive acts or destruction of property" and involve a degree of aggressiveness "grossly out of proportion to any precipitating psychosocial stressors."

IED is a variant of the proverbial "short fuse." Emil Coccaro, the chairman of psychiatry at the University of Chicago is the main expert on IED and coauthored the *Archives* paper. In Coccaro's view, explosive anger is not a normal phenomenon but has its roots in biological variability. I have heard Coccaro suggest at a conference that a basketball coach made famous for assaulting his own players might be a "poster boy" for this diagnosis. IED has also been used in court to defend people accused of acts of criminal violence.

The problem is that *all* variations in human personality and behavior are rooted in biology. Once we start seeing all behavior as biologically determined, there are no limits to the scope of psychiatry. Ironically, this could be a sign that the field is returning to the "bad old days" of psychoanalysis, when we claimed to understand and explain every aspect of human behavior. Psychiatry would no longer be a medical specialty that treats mental disorders but a much vaster enterprise—as much about life as about disease.

The DSM system works better with more severe problems. No one doubts that schizophrenia, mania, and melancholia are dramatically different from normal human experience. But when it comes to the most common conditions in psychiatry (substance abuse, major depression, and many anxiety disorders), the boundaries are not so clear.

All these problems result from the inclusiveness of the DSM philosophy. (I have heard Robert Spitzer say that his priority in developing the DSM-III was to be open to new ideas.) But to put severe mental illnesses in the same category as reactions that are close to normal trivializes psychiatry.

Over time, the number of diagnoses threatens to become almost endless, leading to a serious proliferation of categories. A case in point is that the DSM manual has become much thicker with each edition. It has often been said that people can be divided into those who want to lump many categories of mental illness together, the "lumpers," and those who want to split categories to create new ones, the "splitters." In the DSM, the splitters have run wild, with every piece of the puzzle of mental illness treated as a separate category.

Perhaps the main reason for the large number of diagnoses in psychiatry is that we do not understand any of them. Similar processes of disease may produce symptoms that vary according to the conditions. The large overlap between DSM categories has been misleadingly referred to as "comorbidity," implying that patients have separate disorders (Kessler, Chiu, Demler, Merikangas, & Walters, 2005). But comorbidity is inevitable in a system that separately classifies every variant of illness. Valid diagnosis requires a clear boundary that limits the overlap of one category with neighboring conditions; diagnoses that lack boundaries lack validity.

The Problem of Fuzzy Boundaries

Psychiatrists have always had difficulty establishing a clear cutoff point between pathology and normality because the boundaries of most mental disorders are irredeemably fuzzy. Illness may not form a set of discrete categories but instead be spread across a *spectrum*. There may be some conditions in psychiatry that one either has or does not have. The jury is still out on that issue, but, for example, schizophrenia, classical bipolar disorder, and melancholic depression may be mental illnesses that are either present or absent. However, the most common mental disorders, such as anxiety and depression, have no clear boundary with milder conditions that have some, but not all, of the same features.

One can observe the same problem in medical illnesses. Some infectious diseases (such as measles) are either present or absent. (Even so, we live comfortably with most viruses in our body without falling ill.) In other cases, such as type II diabetes, one sees a continuum. Some patients must take insulin, but there are patients with "pre-diabetes" who could simply prevent the disease by losing weight. Many patients fall between these extremes, and it is not always possible to distinguish overt disease from vulnerability to illness.

In psychiatry, all disorders share some common characteristics. Using a technique called factor analysis, Robert Krueger, a psychologist from the University of Minnesota, has shown that most of the clinical symptoms described by the DSM can be grouped into internalizing disorders (associated with altered mood or anxiety) and externalizing disorders (associated with impulsive actions) (Krueger, 1999). The same groups are commonly used in child psychiatry (where the distinction is even more useful, given that the validity of diagnosis is even more problematic than it is in adults) (Achenbach & McConaughy, 1997).

Many categories of mental illness fall within a spectrum of diagnoses with boundaries that fade into each other, and some lie at the intersection of several spectra. The existence of a *schizophrenic spectrum* (Rosenthal, 1971) is demonstrated by the fact that the relatives of patients with schizophrenia suffer from related conditions (schizotypal and schizoid personality disorders) that show cognitive and interpersonal deficits without the delusions and hallucinations that mark schizophrenia itself (Asarnow et al., 2001). There could be 10 spectrum cases for every diagnosable patient with schizophrenia (Meehl, 1990).

It has also been proposed that there are affective and/or anxiety spectra, an autistic spectrum, and an impulsive spectrum (the latter includes substance abuse, bulimia nervosa, and antisocial and borderline personality disorders) (Jones, Cork, & Chowdhury, 2006; Siever & Davis, 1991; Zanarini, 1993). Chapter 5 will examine the concept of a bipolar spectrum.

These spectra need to be defined through common biological processes and mechanisms. The symptoms of mental disorders are based on more basic mechanisms and pathways (*endophenotypes,* heritable traits or characteristics that are not a direct symptom of a condition but are associated with the underlying processes of disease) (Berrettini, 2005). Thus, endophenotypes may not be visible, unlike the disease itself (the phenotype). Although such processes are more difficult to observe, they are more likely to have biological correlates. If we understood these mechanisms, we could better develop valid diagnoses. (For example, if we had biological markers for schizophrenia, we could determine whether it is one disease or several diseases.)

Moreover, research shows that biological markers have weak or inconsistent relationships with DSM-defined disorders but are more closely related to underlying traits (Nigg, 2006). For example, patients in the schizophrenic spectrum, whether or not they have schizophrenia, tend to have abnormal eye movements (Siever & Davis, 1991). Patients in the impulsive spectrum, independent of diagnosis, tend to have abnormalities in neurochemistry (i.e., decreased brain serotonin activity) and in neurophysiology (i.e., dysfunction in the prefrontal cortex) (Siever & Davis, 1991). These changes are not definite correlates of disease, like an abnormal electrocardiogram. Rather, they are vulnerability markers—like high cholesterol—that may or may not be associated with illness.

These research findings run counter to the approach of the DSM system, in which each category is considered a separate entity. Overlaps and fuzzy boundaries are inevitable if most mental disorders lie on a spectrum (or multiple spectra). However, this concept does not solve the problem of differentiating pathology from normality. We all carry some form of vulnerability, which falls in one spectrum or another. It makes no sense to use a diagnostic system in which almost everyone is considered a potential patient.

Boundary Problems and Social Context

When mental disorders are too broadly defined, their prevalence will be estimated at very high levels. Adding to this problem is the fact that unclear boundaries exist between categories in most of the diagnoses in the DSM system.

Mood disorders provide many examples of this problem (see Chapter 5), but substance abuse, as defined in the DSM, offers an even more striking illustration. In a survey that used DSM-III criteria, about 10% of men in America were found to meet the diagnostic criteria for alcoholism (Robins & Regier, 1991). This is an enormously high prevalence. The number might be valid, but it might also reflect the failure of DSM criteria to distinguish between excessive drinking and addictive disease. How much do you have to drink, and how much does drinking have to affect your life, before you are considered an alcoholic? There is no obvious way to draw such a definitive boundary. Although we can assess addiction by the presence of withdrawal symptoms, such as delirium tremens, it is much more difficult to know precisely what constitutes alcohol abuse. We are looking at a continuum—the more one drinks, the worse the consequences. Substance use has been ubiquitous throughout human history. Yet not everyone who abuses substances needs to be considered as having a mental disorder. For consistency, nicotine dependence was listed in the DSM. Because tobacco is a substance that kills people, we might consider addiction to it as being as serious as alcoholism. But, in practice, nobody does. To be even *more* consistent, we might also include dependence on caffeine (another highly addictive substance, which may not cause dysfunction but does cause withdrawal symptoms). Just imagine what a large proportion of the population might meet criteria for a mental disorder if we were to extend the boundaries in that way.

Social phobia is a diagnosis that raises similar problems (Wakefield, Horwitz, & Schmitz, 2005). This category describes patients who suffer from anxiety when in unfamiliar social situations. Many people experience this kind of problem, particularly when having to speak in public or attend a party where they do not know anyone. (There is some evidence that antidepressants help reduce social anxiety [Wakefield, 2005].) But there is no clear boundary between social phobia and shyness. Social phobia is one end of a normal range of variation. Many people with these symptoms work their way around them. Social phobia is certainly not a disease that produces consistent dysfunction in the same sense that mental disorders such as schizophrenia do.

Autism is much in the news these days. But the boundaries of this disorder have now been extended to include a spectrum of conditions falling within the overall group "pervasive developmental disorders" (Szatmari, 2004). Children and adults with Asperger's syndrome have milder symptoms (impaired social interaction and stereotyped behaviors) that resemble autism. However, the syndrome's separation from normality remains unclear. Does every nerd have Asperger's? Some people have a tendency to prefer *things* to other people yet manage to function in life. At what point should this pattern be considered an autistic spectrum disorder?

Human beings show wide variations in behavior, thought, and emotion. The effects of individual differences depend on context. In most situations, these variations are harmless. For example, social drinking is more attractive to some people than to others, even if inebriation has existed since grapes were first harvested. Shy people are not necessarily disordered if they find a way of life that suits them. The issue that is being ignored is social context (Paris, 1996). Many disorders in psychiatry are much more (or less) prevalent in one society than in another. They reflect traits that serve one well in some social settings and badly in others. The main exceptions are severe illnesses such as schizophrenia and bipolar disorder, which are universal and cause dysfunction in any person, whatever the context. Milder forms of illness are less likely to be universal.

Conclusion

Psychiatric diagnoses cannot be assumed to describe diseases in the same way that diagnoses in other branches of medicine can. The underlying processes behind mental illness remain to be discovered. Moreover, symptoms of mental illness can be shaped by psychological adversities and by social context. Until we learn more from research about the biological nature of mental disorders and about the impact of the environment on this biology, our categories will inevitably have fuzzy boundaries. In the meantime, we need to remember that although diagnosis is a necessary tool of the trade, the tools in the DSM should not be reified. And we need to keep in mind that although all variants of behavior have biological correlates, they need not be classified as mental disorders.

5

Mood and Mental Illness

Depression and Unhappiness

Depression is a state of mind that most people can understand on some level. Most of us experience periods of sadness or grief after losses or disappointments in life, and some of us know what it is like to be unhappy for months, or even years at a time. But at what point does depressed mood become a mental disorder? Unfortunately, the broad concept used in contemporary psychiatry fails to answer this question and to distinguish between normal unhappiness, an experience not uncommon in everyday life, and the paralyzing disorder that is clinical depression.

The DSM does allow for extended periods of symptomatic distress following bereavement but does not apply this principle to other losses. A recent study showed that the prevalence of depression in the community would be much lower if we were to exclude syndromes arising from stressors that occur more frequently (and normally) in the community (Wakefield, Schmitz, First, & Horwitz, 2007). Freud (1957) had an interesting take on this problem, noting with irony (and honesty) that all his treatment aimed to do was turn neurotic misery into normal human unhappiness.

Although now it seems that no one is able to define this boundary, this was not always the case. Years ago, psychiatrists treated incapacitating depressions in the mental hospital, where only the sickest patients were seen. But once psychiatry began to be practiced in offices, practitioners started seeing patients with milder symptoms. With the introduction of the DSM-III and its successors, psychiatry widened its net to diagnose as depression many states of mind marked by distress and psychological suffering.

Depression has been defined differently from one era to the next. In the era of mental hospitals, it was often limited to *melancholia*. That term, which dates back to Hippocrates, describes a condition lasting weeks to months in which patients suffer from despondency, irritability, and restlessness, with a slowing down of mental processes and movement, and diminished appetite, sleeplessness, and powerful suicidal urges (Parker, 2005a, 2005b). Melancholia is probably one of the few psychiatric conditions that is much like a medical disease. And melancholic depression responds fairly specifically to treatment methods, particularly tricyclic antidepressants and electroconvulsive therapy (Parker, 2005a, 2005b).

In contrast, "major depressive disorder" in the DSM-IV-TR has little resemblance to a medical diagnosis (Parker & Manicavasagar, 2005). This disorder requires that 5 of 9 listed symptoms be present: (1) depressed mood, (2) diminished interest or pleasure in activities, (3) weight loss or weight gain, (4) insomnia or hypersomnia, (5) agitation or motor retardation, (6) fatigue or loss of energy, (7) feelings of worthlessness or guilt, (8) diminished concentration, (9) suicidal ideation (American Psychiatric Association, 2000). (The DSM manual also requires that one of the first two be present.)

The more severe subtypes of depression are defined more narrowly than is major depression. The DSM allows us to code depression by severity, presence of melancholic features, or presence of psychotic symptoms, such as delusions. Also, the manual requires that depression affect functioning "significantly" (although anyone with 5 criteria would be significantly affected in some way).

In practice, even when mildly depressed, many people meet 5 of 9 listed criteria. It is not clear why the number required for diagnosis is 5, and not 6, 7, or 8. A more troubling detail in the definition is the minimum length of time required to make a diagnosis of major depression: only two weeks. In the course of a lifetime, how many of us have suffered from continuous low mood for a couple of weeks? Not to feel this way after losing a job or a lover, for example, might actually be abnormal. On the other hand, milder depressions, lasting for short periods, are often triggered by losses of that kind. Although the DSM specifically allows that normal bereavement go on for longer than a few weeks, it fails to specify the same principle for other losses precipitating depression (Kendler, Neale, & Kessler, 1995). The crucial point is that the time frame in the DSM (2 weeks) makes it almost impossible to separate depression from grief and loss.

Thus, what the DSM calls "major depression" is often not really that "major." But the manual's use of this terminology has misled psychiatrists into believing that the experience of depression, largely regardless of context, is a disease no different from those treated by other physicians.

The origins of the DSM system's broad definition of depression date back more than 30 years. A highly influential article by Hagop Akiskal and William McKinney suggested that older distinctions between types of depression did not fit data indicating that all depressions lie on a continuum (Akiskal & McKinney, 1973). Previous classifications had distinguished between "garden-variety" depressions (formerly called "depressive neuroses") and more severe types (melancholic or psychotic depression) (American Psychiatric Association, 1968). But all depressions, from the mildest to the most severe, have symptoms in common. Moreover, Akiskal and McKinney pointed out that there was no evidence that mild depression is purely environmental, or that severe depression is purely biological. If the same causes can lead to mild or to severe impairment, no basis exists for dividing depression into separate categories. Another argument in favor of a unitary theory was that relatives of patients with severe depression may develop only milder forms of the illness.

Most experts on mood disorders were impressed by Akiskal and McKinney's arguments. In the DSM-III, all subtypes were included within the broad category of major depressive disorder. Over time the unitary approach to depression became conventional wisdom. All the same, the concept remains open to challenge.

Depressed mood is a symptom, like inflammation, that can produce similar effects in many different diseases. It is legitimate to ask whether melancholic depression, a condition in which patients cannot function at all, and which sees 10% of sufferers commit suicide, is really the same disorder as a low mood lasting for a few weeks (Parker & Manicavasagar, 2005). Because people with milder depressions also suffer, they have good reasons to seek treatment. Yet to describe brief episodes of sadness, during which patients often continue to function, as being on a continuum with melancholia, in which they cannot function, is questionable. Although the unitary theory of depression might be vindicated in the end, we need much more evidence before we can accept it. Once again, psychiatry suffers from having no blood tests or other biological markers to establish the boundaries of its diagnostic categories.

The practical problem with a unitary diagnosis of major depression is that it primes psychiatrists to treat most depressed patients with drugs. (Even the term "major" seems to push us to do something, rather than merely stand by.) Although this was not the intention of the DSM, the reification of the diagnosis has led psychiatrists to believe that it would be wrong not to offer pharmacotherapy. It has also led us to forget the importance of psychotherapy, which is known to be an effective treatment for depression.

In fact, the milder and less typical forms of major depression do not always respond to treatment in the same way. As Chapter 8 will show, not every depressed patient responds to antidepressants. Drugs are most effective for severe depression, and much less useful for episodes of lowered mood related to the vicissitudes of life. Moreover, patients may have problems beyond mood disorders (such as addictions or personality disorders) that make them less likely to respond to drugs.

The idea that major depression is a unique disease requiring unique treatment is an oversimplification of a very complex issue. In most of the patients psychiatrists treat, depression is either a syndrome or only a symptom. Depressed patients may respond to antidepressants, to psychotherapy alone, or to a combination of both (Klerman, DiMascio, Weissman, Prusoff, & Paykel, 1974). Each case is different, and psychiatrists must take these differences into account.

How Prevalent Is Depression?

Depression has been called the common cold of psychiatry. As presently defined, it seems to have been increasing in prevalence over recent decades and can affect an even larger proportion of people over a lifetime (Goldberg, 2006). But this statement presumes that all depressions are one disorder, confusing mild with severe cases and running the risk of trivializing melancholia, a dangerous and disabling illness. Such definitional problems thus affect how accurately we can measure the prevalence of depression in the general population. Estimates of lifetime rates of depression have been variable as a result—with some as high as 20% (Waraich, Goldner, Somers, & Hsu, 2004). Major depression is also more common in women than in men, making the proportion of depressed women even higher (Goldberg, 2006). To cite another example, the National Comorbidity Survey, the large-scale United States epidemiological study that made use of DSM criteria for major depression, determined that the lifetime prevalence of the disorder is 16.6%—that is, one out of six people will suffer a major depression sometime in his or her life (Kessler, Chiu, Demler, Merikangas, & Walters, 2005). Is this estimate credible, or should we consider whether it is an artifact of how the DSM defines the disorder?

Depression, however broadly defined, nevertheless *does* present an important public health problem. The World Health Organization (WHO) has published research on the global burden of disease, in a study whose main purpose was to determine the causes of poor health in various regions of the world (Lopez, Mathers, Ezzati, Jamison, & Murray, 2006). To that end, WHO examined data on the effect of various diseases on occupational and social functioning, and on mortality. The project then calculated a measure called total "disability adjusted life years" (DALYs). The results showed that depression was the fourth leading cause of disease burden, accounting for 3.7% of all DALYs in the world.

The effect of depression on general health should come as no surprise to psychiatrists and family doctors, who see patients with these problems every day. If there was anything unexpected about the WHO report, it was the fact that depression was ranked as causing more disability than any other illness except lung infections, gastrointestinal infections, and the complications of childbirth. Thus the global burden of disease is greater for depression than for known killers such as tuberculosis, malaria, heart disease, stroke, and cancer.

Nonetheless, the effects of depression on health might be largely due to the impact of the most severe cases. The WHO study did not examine this possibility, even though it seems likely to be a major factor.

Depressions lasting a few weeks, which are not severe enough to stop people from working or socializing, may not be associated with long-term disability. And although a predisposition to depression may express itself in more or less severe ways, that does not prove that all forms are equivalent (Akiskal & McKinney, 1973).

A greater concern is how these theories play out in practice. As depression has become *reified*, psychiatrists have come to regard it as a disease entity rather than as a useful label. Yet there are many ways to be depressed, and pervasive sadness is seen in many diagnostic categories. It may indeed be worthwhile to treat patients who do not have classical symptoms by prescribing an antidepressant, but that strategy is not consistently successful (see Chapter 8).

The unitary theory of depression has led psychiatry and the DSM system to define this group of disorders inclusively. Hence, depression, to whatever degree, is considered a single disease that can be said to affect hundreds of millions of people worldwide. This alarmingly high prevalence of disorder, however, depends on assumptions that pathologize the human condition and do not reflect solid science.

Chronic Depression and Personality Disorders

Depression is an abnormal but usually temporary state of mind. Lowered mood may last for weeks or months, but most people eventually return to normal. On the other hand, depression is, in a fair percentage of cases, a recurrent disease (Goldberg, 2006). Some people never fully recover and remain chronically depressed.

Cases in which depression is chronic are widely recognized but often viewed through the lens of the unitary theory as a disease variant. When patients develop a serious depression and never seem to be quite well thereafter, they may meet criteria for a milder type of mood disorder called dysthymia. To meet the DSM-IV-TR criteria for that condition, patients need to have only two symptoms in addition to depressed mood present for more days than not for a period of at least two years (American Psychiatric Association, 2000).

Dysthymia is not a unitary diagnosis (Klein & Santiago, 2003; Niculescu & Akiskal, 2001). Some patients develop these symptoms because they never recover from a serious bout of acute depression, whereas patients who have never had acute episodes become and remain chronically depressed. One reason for chronic depression can be that the life of a patient is objectively unhappy. And that is more likely to occur when the patient has personality problems that lead to bad choices in work and relationships.

Personality disorder is an important concept in psychiatry (Paris, 2003, 2005b). It describes conditions characterized by problems in mood, behavior, thought, interpersonal relationships, and impulse control that occur in a wide range of situations, lead to significant dysfunction, start early in life, and continue for many years.

But psychiatrists have a certain resistance to making these diagnoses (Lewis & Appleby, 1988). Practitioners like to focus on what they can treat, and many see personality disorders as not very treatable. In point of fact, most patients with such disorders *are* treatable, just not necessarily through medication. That said, such patients are certainly a challenge, and many do present symptoms of depression and anxiety that can confuse the clinical picture.

Dysthymia during adolescence is a marker for the development of personality disorders (Pepper et al., 1995). Also, many patients with these diagnoses have periods when they meet criteria for major depression. For this reason, psychiatrists may be tempted to see them narrowly as just "cases" of depression (or of "treatment-resistant depression") and to prescribe them antidepressants. However, research suggests that these are exactly the people who often fail to respond, or only partially respond, to drugs (Newton-Howes, Tyrer, & Johnson, 2006; Shea et al., 1990, 1992). Although drugs take the edge off the mood disturbance in these patients, one does not see remission (Paris, 2005b). And when results are not good, psychiatrists are tempted to try even harder; consequently, the patient can end up on multiple drugs, none of which turns out to be dramatically effective (Zanarini, Frankenburg, Khera, & Bleichmar, 2001).

Psychiatry's reification of depression and its obsession with pharmacology can lead to bad treatment, and this has especially been the case with personality disorders. These are complex conditions for which we now have several effective psychotherapeutic methods (Paris, 2005b). It should be emphasized that most of the research on these methods concerns borderline personality disorder—patients who are chronically suicidal, repeatedly cut themselves for relief of distress, and have very disturbed relationships. In these cases especially, prescribing drugs alone can sometimes be counterproductive.

I might be accused of being self-serving in trying to convince my colleagues to give more consideration to personality disorders—the conditions I have spent my life studying. But these diagnoses describe a rich range of symptoms, including the life problems that psychiatrists have traditionally treated—not a narrow range of symptoms that can be easily targeted with drugs. These are the kind of symptoms that have always required skilled psychotherapy, even if drugs play some role in management. In short, seeing everything in psychiatry as related to mood is bad medicine.

Bipolar Disorder

Of all the categories in the DSM, the one that is currently most seriously over-diagnosed is bipolar disorder. Again, the problem involves distinguishing among serious mental disorders, milder problems, and normal variations in mood. Many people are moody. Quite a few of us experience ups and downs. Only recently has it become fashionable to consider these mood variations features of bipolarity.

Bipolar disorder is a new name for an old disease. In the nineteenth century, mental illnesses were divided into psychoses (which affected the appreciation of reality) and neuroses (which did not). A hundred years ago, the German psychiatrist Emil Kraepelin (1856–1926) divided the psychoses into two large groups—one that affected thought and had a steadily deteriorating course, and one that affected mood and had an intermittent course (Kraepelin, 1921). The first type was called dementia praecox, later renamed schizophrenia; the second was manic-depression, later renamed bipolar disorder.

Schizophrenia is a term introduced by the Swiss psychiatrist Eugen Bleuler (1857–1939) (Bleuler, 1950). This disorder is marked by abnormal thought patterns, delusions, and hallucinations. Patients usually have an early onset of psychosis, are never fully well thereafter, and go steadily downhill. In contrast, manic-depression mainly affects mood (causing it to be either too high or too low), and delusions and hallucinations are seen only at the height of manic or depressive phases. Thus, most bipolar patients tend to have an episodic illness with periods of normality between episodes.

This separation became even more important when it was found that drugs affect each condition differently. Schizophrenia is treated with antipsychotic drugs, which can also prevent relapses. Bipolar disorder also responds to antipsychotic drugs, but the relapse rate and the course of the disorder are unaffected.

Lithium, a salt that was first used in 1949 by the Australian psychiatrist John Cade to treat mania, allowed psychiatrists to prevent recurrences of mania for the first time. But the drug was initially shelved because of concerns about its toxicity. The revival of interest in lithium started with the research of the Danish psychiatrist Mogens Schou (1918–2005). Schou (2001) began to use lithium as early as 1952, but it took him another 15 years to prove its efficacy. Once the research group demonstrated lithium's value for preventing recurrences of bipolar illness, lithium began to be prescribed widely all over the world.

I was a psychiatric resident at the time lithium was introduced, and I still consider this drug to be the greatest medical miracle I have seen. I was the first physician at my hospital to prescribe it. The drug was so new we had to order it from an outside pharmacy. The patient we were treating at the time was a woman who had been hospitalized more than 20 times and treated with antipsychotics (with only temporary effects). Once on lithium, she was never hospitalized again. I felt as if I had been present at the first administration of penicillin.

Lithium is still the drug that has been most documented to prevent recurrence of bipolar disorder (Taylor & Goodwin, 2006). Some research suggests that patients who take lithium are less likely to commit suicide than those who do not (Goodwin et al., 2003). Given the 10% suicide rate associated with bipolar illness, this is an important advantage. Unfortunately, lithium is rather toxic, and its use must be monitored closely because it can cause kidney and thyroid problems. It has as a result suffered the fate of many effective drugs in medicine in that it has been supplanted by the "new kids on the block"—anticonvulsants used as mood stabilizers (valproate, topiramate, lamotrigine)—which have fewer side effects than lithium does. There is, however, less evidence that these newer agents are effective in preventing recurrences of mania (Goodwin & Jamison, 2007).

Why Bipolar Disorder Is Over-Diagnosed

Psychiatrists found that some of their most difficult patients benefited from lithium. In fact, many patients who had been diagnosed with schizophrenia were now seen as bipolar because of their response to the drug. This very responsiveness thus became a benchmark for other changes in diagnosis from schizophrenia to bipolar disorder. And yet the distinction between the two is still not always clear. Kraepelin's original division, however much it revolutionized psychiatry, remains controversial (Goodwin & Jamison, 2007). Typical cases of schizophrenia and bipolar disorder do not create any diagnostic problems, but some patients seem to fall on the boundary between the categories. Moreover, many patients with bipolar disorder fail to show the intermittent periods of recovery that are considered a hallmark of that illness. Recent research has blurred the lines even more by suggesting that psychotic symptoms in both conditions may be influenced by the same genes and shaped by a common neurobiology (McInnis et al., 2003).

This research demonstrates (once again) that psychiatrists do not know enough to make specific diagnoses through biological markers— neither genes nor laboratory findings are of help at this point. We remain dependent on signs and symptoms, but observation alone cannot clarify the boundaries of mental disorders, even of those that are severe. Are psychoses single diseases or many diseases? We still do not know.

Ironically, before the introduction of lithium, we over-diagnosed schizophrenia. Forty to fifty years ago, patients who were a little strange, or just lonely, were often seen as suffering from "latent schizophrenia," "ambulatory schizophrenia," or "pseudo-neurotic schizophrenia" (multiple neurotic symptoms thought to reflect an underlying schizophrenic process) (Hoch, Cattell, Strahl, & Penness, 1962). Some of these patients may have fallen within a "schizophrenic spectrum" (milder conditions that do not go on to psychosis). Most, however, were likely misdiagnosed—victims of a diagnostic fad that, in the absence of established markers for disease, ran unchecked for many years.

Difficulty distinguishing the two conditions seemed also to fall along national lines. Research in the early 1970s showed, for example, that U.S. psychiatrists were diagnosing schizophrenia in patients whom British psychiatrists considered to be suffering from bipolar disorder (Cooper, Kendell, & Gurland, 1972). This landmark study, which showed videotaped interviews of the same patients to psychiatrists in New York and London and documented how each group arrived at different diagnostic conclusions, led many to reexamine their diagnostic practices, especially once diagnosis made a difference in treatment. Indeed, until the introduction of lithium, it did not matter that much which diagnosis psychotic patients received. The only medications available were antipsychotic drugs, which achieved symptom control in both conditions. For manic patients, the antipsychotics had only a brief calming effect, after which many patients inevitably relapsed. Once lithium proved effective at preventing recurrences, however, accurate diagnosis became crucial for the management of bipolar patients.

Thus, the New York–London study occurred at about the time when psychiatrists realized that lithium was indeed an effective and specific treatment for mania. In the 1970s the hope of curing psychotic patients with lithium was gaining significant momentum, backed by Schou's efficacy research. What followed was a dramatic decrease in the frequency of the diagnosis of schizophrenia and a rethinking of it in terms of the diagnosis of bipolar disorder. For example, two psychiatrists at the University of Chicago, Richard Abrams and Michael Taylor (1981), examined many of the classical features of schizophrenia described by European psychiatrists (such as delusions involving the idea of thought control) and found that such symptoms are equally common in bipolar patients. Abrams and Taylor subsequently rediagnosed as manic-depressive many of their patients who had previously been called schizophrenic—to such an extent that schizophrenia became a rare disease on their unit.

Thus was born the fad of over-diagnosing bipolar disorder. Some psychiatrists, faced with a psychotic patient, now preferred to make a diagnosis of bipolar disorder because they believed it has a better prognosis than does schizophrenia (although this is not always the case). In fact, that belief is emblematic of a larger tendency in the field to believe that a treatment effective for one condition (in this case, lithium for bipolar disorder) can be used effectively for all conditions. This is typical in psychiatry. From psychoanalysis to electroconvulsive therapy, treatments that help *some* patients have been prescribed to almost everyone else, on the off chance that they might work. It is all too easy to "shoehorn" patients into diagnoses to justify these therapies.

Thus, whereas some patients who had been misdiagnosed with schizophrenia were correctly redefined as suffering from bipolar disorder (and responded with gratifying success to lithium), many others who had been diagnosed correctly as schizophrenic were tried on this drug with minimal justification and little success. Any sign of depression in schizophrenic patients would be pounced on as proof that they "really" suffered from a mood disorder. Agitated psychotic states were routinely defined as manic episodes. Even in the most chronic cases of schizophrenia, psychiatrists have used the "fudge" diagnosis of "schizo-affective disorder" (a mixture of schizophrenia and manic-depression) to justify prescribing lithium. For a time, it was almost impossible to leave a hospital ward without receiving a lithium prescription. And because patients tend to get better after *any* hospitalization, psychiatrists interpreted such improvements as clinical responses. The result was that many patients were unnecessarily and ineffectively kept on lithium for years afterward.

Some psychiatrists are reluctant to "deny patients the benefit" of lithium, but the benefit is illusory if the patients do not in fact have bipolar disorder. And continuing to prescribe it in the absence of any clear benefit at the very least communicates a false hope—especially to patients with schizophrenia and to their families—that can be worse than no hope at all. We do patients and their families no favors by misleading them about a diagnosis, however tragic it may be, and about its treatments. We owe them instead our commitment to helping them manage their illness and to offering them treatments, be they antipsychotics or psychotherapy or psychiatric rehabilitation (or all of these), that have been proven in cases similar to theirs to enhance the management of their illness.

A few years ago, I was interviewed by a local reporter who took the opportunity to share with me his bitterness about the condition of his mentally ill sister: In spite of being diagnosed with and treated for bipolar disorder, she continued to be psychotic and decline. I could not tell him that I had seen his sister in consultation some years before and had had little doubt that the correct diagnosis was schizophrenia. Although not every patient with that diagnosis deteriorates, this incident speaks to the limits of false hope when one is treated for an illness one does not have instead of for the illness one does.

Bipolar Imperialism

Over-diagnosis of bipolar disorder did not stop with the reclassification of psychoses. It went on to include patients with a number of other problems that had little to do with psychosis (or with the traditional concept of manic-depression) (Ghaemi, Ko, & Goodwin, 2002). A broader diagnosis of bipolar disorder was eventually proposed, based on ideas that are not built on biological benchmarks but that co-opt several other traditionally separate diagnoses (Goodwin & Ghaemi, 2003). The result: Unipolar depression, addictions, personality disorders, and behavioral disturbances in children have all been seen as forms of bipolarity (Judd et al., 2003). I like to call this *bipolar imperialism.*

There are many reasons for the emergence of this diagnostic fad. But the idea that all mood instability is a symptom of bipolar illness is the driving concept. According to this concept, classical manic-depression is the severe end of a continuum, with milder conditions called "bipolar spectrum disorders" occurring toward the other end of that continuum.

Other reasons for bipolar imperialism include the systematic marketing of the diagnosis by pharmaceutical companies making mood stabilizers. Another factor is the (incorrect) belief that bipolar disorder is more treatable than are other conditions. And still another factor is psychiatrists' wishes to manage difficult patients (such as those with substance abuse and personality disorders) by redefining them as having a treatable chemical imbalance.

Mania is an unmistakable state. Patients are excited, talk and think very rapidly, and may not need sleep for days or weeks. They can spend money wildly, make countless long-distance phone calls, and buy multiple cars or other expensive items in quantity. However, some patients have milder forms of the illness, in which one sees "hypomanic" rather than "manic" episodes. In hypomania, people continue to function; those in full mania cannot. Another difference is the time frame: Mania can last for weeks (or even months), whereas hypomania may last only a few days.

To account for patients who never have full manic episodes, a new diagnosis emerged, bipolar II disorder, to be distinguished from bipolar I disorder (classical manic depression) (Judd et al., 2003). Patients with bipolar II have mood swings that range only from depression to hypomania. I have seen many such patients and agree that this is indeed a milder form of bipolar I. Otherwise well functioning, people with bipolar II can have brief "high" periods, lasting for days to weeks, in which they feel increased energy and indulge impulses, such as overspending.

As is generally true of psychiatric diagnosis, those cases that are most severe produce the clearest and most valid categories, whereas less severe cases overlap with other disorders (or with normality). The diagnosis of bipolar II should not be given to anyone with mood swings—they must have had full-blown hypomanic episodes (which require a continuous "high" for at least four days). Mood swings that last a few hours to a day or so are more characteristic of personality disorders, conditions that do not evolve into bipolar illness or respond to the same forms of treatment (Paris, Gunderson, & Weinberg, 2007).

In fact, there may be two groups of patients currently being diagnosed as having bipolar II. One falls within the bipolar spectrum, the other does not. One responds well to the same mood stabilizers that are used for bipolar I, and one does not.

If bipolar II were diagnosed rigorously, there would not be a problem; however, clinicians have been interpreting mood swings of all kinds as a marker for the condition. This is probably why patients meeting criteria for bipolar II tend to have relatives with a wide variety of other conditions (Paris, Gunderson, & Weinberg, 2007). And the likelihood that bipolar II is being over-diagnosed helps explain its treatment response—many patients who receive the diagnosis do not consistently respond to the drugs that are used (more effectively) in bipolar I (Paris, Gunderson, & Weinberg, 2007).

Another point of confusion is the idea that one can see "mixed states" of mania and depression in patients who do not have hypomanic episodes (Akiskal, 2002; Angst & Gamma, 2002). The problem with this somewhat slippery concept is that it can be used to describe all kinds of abnormal states of mind, even in patients who never have consistently elevated moods.

In spite of the problems with establishing the boundaries of bipolar II disorder, several experts have proposed that psychiatry should adopt an even wider spectrum. These research groups (led by Hagop Akiskal in San Diego, Fred Goodwin in Washington, DC, and Jules Angst in Zurich, Switzerland) all want to expand bipolar disorders to encompass other conditions (Akiskal, 2002; Angst & Gamma, 2002; Ghaemi et al., 2002). In this schema, bipolarity could take four basic forms: *bipolar I,* the classical manic-depressive diagnosis described by Kraepelin; *bipolar II,* depression with spontaneous hypomanic episodes; *bipolar III,* in which hypomanic episodes occur only as a result of taking antidepressants; and *bipolar IV,* an "ultra-rapid-cycling" disorder in which mood swings occur on a daily or even hourly basis (Ghaemi et al., 2002).

Epidemiological research suggests that bipolar I and bipolar II disorder combined are present in about 2–4% of the population (Kessler et al., 1994). If we were to adopt a concept of "soft bipolarity," in which most depressions, substance abuse, personality disorders, and childhood behavioral disorders were seen as "really" bipolar, the total prevalence could reach 10% or more (Angst & Gamma, 2002). Such a dramatic increase might raise the question (as framed by my colleague Scott Patten (2006) in a debate published in the *Canadian Journal of Psychiatry*): "Is There Anyone Who *Doesn't* Have Bipolar Disorder?"

In fact, bipolar imperialism aims to take over much of psychiatry; its proponents want to treat large numbers of patients with mood stabilizers. But unstable mood, like depression, is a symptom, not a disease. It alone does not point to any one diagnosis or any one form of treatment. The symptom of mood shifting from day to day, or even from hour to hour, in response to life events (a condition that has been called "affective instability" or "emotional dysregulation") is characteristic of borderline personality disorder (Henry et al., 2001; Linehan, 1993; Siever & Davis, 1991). To the bipolar imperialists, however, such an argument is unconvincing. They believe that diagnoses like personality disorder do not exist but are simply points along the bipolar spectrum.

As a consultant, I have to deal with the effects of the "mania" for diagnosing bipolar disorder. Every patient with unstable mood (and there are many) will be sent to me for assessment with a note from the referring physician asking, "Is this bipolar disorder?" And patients themselves (or their spouses, partners, and relatives) come in asking if moodiness implies this diagnosis. If their mood is unstable, are they are "really" bipolar? Now regularly confronted with such questions, my first response is to ask whether the patient has ever been hospitalized. Since true mania almost always requires hospitalization, patients who have never been admitted are unlikely to have had this condition.

Bipolar imperialism has also attracted biographers and historians. Of course, making historical diagnoses breaks a standard rule of medicine— not to categorize people you have never met. Nonetheless, Kay Jamison (1993), a research psychologist (who herself suffers from bipolar I disorder), has published a book claiming that many famous people in history have had this condition. Other historical diagnoses of bipolarity have been made for Abraham Lincoln, Winston Churchill, and Nikita

Khrushchev.[1] One recent book even claimed that Lyndon Johnson suffered from this disorder, leading to the Vietnam War (Jablow, 2002). Bipolar imperialism is madness with real consequences. Because there is little evidence that unstable mood (as opposed to hypomania or mania) responds to the same treatments that stabilize classical manic-depression, many patients will get the wrong diagnosis and the wrong treatment. Bipolar imperialism has led thousands to receive drugs they do not need. This is a development that the pharmaceutical industry in the United States has strongly encouraged, more so now than ever before in that it is allowed to advertise directly to the public. For example, Astra-Zeneca, which produces the antipsychotic Seroquel (quetiapine), which was recently approved for the treatment of bipolar disorder, sponsors ads linking consumers to a Web site called "isitreallydepression.com." The company aims to convince people who feel depressed that they could really be suffering from bipolar illness. They list a number of "soft signs" of mania, such as periods of elevated mood, irritability, increased energy, and increased spending. Although it is true that such symptoms, if severe, could point to mania, most occur from time to time in normal people. But the real purpose of the advertisement was to encourage people to take drugs (particularly the one that AstraZeneca manufactures).

Not everyone is convinced that drugs are the right treatment choice or even that bipolar disorder is the right diagnosis. In 2004 *New York Magazine* published a cover story entitled "Are You Bipolar?" that described how a large number of patients, even those with mild mood swings, are being given this diagnosis and treated with the drugs developed for classical cases (Grigoriadis, 2004). The author of the article, who had been diagnosed as bipolar, went on to describe how she gained more from psychotherapy than from any of the drugs (with their numerous side effects) that had been prescribed for her.

Bipolar Disorder and Childhood

The concept that childhood behavioral disorders are forms of bipolar illness raises another serious concern about diagnosis. Since the time of Kraepelin, psychiatrists have believed that mania begins no earlier than adolescence. The proposal that it can start in childhood, before puberty, is new (Duffy, 2007).

The idea of childhood bipolarity depends on a further expansion of the definition of mood instability to include irritability and anger. Although it is true that some patients with mania and hypomania do not describe feeling "high" (i.e., do not have grandiose ideas or act in ways that suggest they are invincible or on top of the world) but instead say they mainly feel irritable, continuous irritability and anger do not necessarily point to a bipolar diagnosis (Abrams & Taylor, 1981). They are common symptoms that are associated with many other psychological problems.

In children, for example, aggressive behavior and emotional dysregulation were, in the past, usually diagnosed as symptomatic of conduct disorder, a condition that is associated with aggression and delinquency and that is a frequent precursor of criminality and/or antisocial personality in adulthood (Kazdin, 1996). Less severe behavioral problems were diagnosed as oppositional defiant disorder. And many behavioral problems in childhood can be understood as a consequence of attention-deficit hyperactivity disorder (ADHD), a category to be discussed in more detail in Chapter 6.

To see children with such behavioral problems as suffering from bipolar disorder implies a more serious prognosis (children with conduct disorder may improve over time). It also leads to the prescription of one or several drugs to control behaviors that are seen as symptoms of bipolarity. Yet there are no biological markers that we can use to confirm whether in fact these children warrant this diagnosis.

No one can deny that children with these problems are difficult to manage and that their behavior is of great concern to their families. Their prognosis is also of concern. We have data showing that such problems tend to persist in adolescence, but that does not prove that they are indications of bipolarity (Birmayer et al., 2006). Nor has it yet been shown that children with mood instability and impulsive behaviors actually develop bipolar disorder later in life.

It is faddish to view almost every childhood behavioral problem as evidence of a mood disorder, and it is worrying that such a view has resulted in large numbers of children being prescribed mood stabilizers and antipsychotic drugs (Olfson, Blanco, Liu, Moreno, & Laje, 2006). These concerns have now been widely circulated in the media. Although these drugs have a calming effect that reduces aggression in impulsive children, there are many other ways to achieve the same goal.

Meanwhile, patients who receive these agents can expect to be on them for many years—if not for life. This could turn out to be one of the worst scandals in the history of psychiatry—and we have had quite a few.

Conclusion

Psychiatrists have to understand a bewildering range of phenomena and symptoms in their patients. Life would be simpler if these problems were all the result of chemical imbalances and abnormal mood, for then we could treat everyone with drugs, and our success would depend only on our skill in mixing and matching these agents.

But life is not simple, and most mental health conditions are not easily understood from signs and symptoms alone. To think that they can be is an example of the dangers of reductionism and has led to misguided treatment methods in psychiatry.

One measure is the dramatic increase in antidepressant prescriptions over the last decade (Paulose-Ram, Safran, Jonas, Gu, & Orwig, in press; Raymond, Morgan, & Caetano, 2007). A large-scale survey in the United States, for example, found that the proportion of treated individuals who used antidepressant medications increased from 37% to 75%, whereas the proportion who received any form of psychotherapy declined from 71% to 60% (Olfson et al., 2002). Even though drugs for the treatment of mood disorders are not consistently effective, experts are promoting the view that antidepressants and mood stabilizers are the main (or even the only) answer to depression and overly reactive mood. This is simply untrue and can only harm the reputation of psychiatry.

6

Psychiatry's Problem Children

M ood disorders are only one of the controversial diagnoses in modern psychiatry. Attention-deficit hyperactivity disorder (ADHD), post-traumatic stress disorder (PTSD), dissociative disorders, and personality disorders can be described as psychiatry's "problem children." Some of these diagnostic categories are valid, and some are not. All of them can be over-diagnosed.

The Boundaries of ADHD

ADHD is a diagnosis that has aroused public controversy, especially given that the standard treatment is to administer stimulant medication. Some people find the very idea of medicating children to be troubling, and in certain circumstances, such as those discussed in the previous chapter, over-prescription has indeed been a problem. But several critics of psychiatry have seized on this issue as part of their attack on the whole discipline. Every year at the American Psychiatric Association's annual meeting, for example, demonstrators (sponsored by the Church of Scientology) conduct a noisy demonstration for TV cameras in front of the convention center, accusing psychiatrists of "drugging kids." They are objecting to medicating what, to them, is an invented diagnosis: ADHD. But ADHD is a real disorder, and typical cases are unmistakable. Children with this diagnosis show three clinical characteristics— overactivity, distractability, and impulsivity. In classical ADHD, all these symptoms respond well to medications such as methylphenidate (Ritalin) (Wender, 2000). The problem is that not every diagnosed case of ADHD is "classical," and many children do not respond to standard stimulant medication (Biederman, 2005; Leung & Lemay, 2003). The most likely explanation for this circumstance is that ADHD has fuzzy boundaries.

There is no blood test or brain scan that can tell you whether a patient does or does not have ADHD. Diagnosis is based on observations of behavior that can often be subjective, guided by DSM-IV criteria that are themselves imprecise. And when the boundaries are fuzzy, over-diagnosis becomes a danger. A tip-off that this has occurred with ADHD is its high prevalence: Estimates vary, but some have suggested that 10% of all boys have been diagnosed with it (Rowland, Lesesne, & Abramowitz, 2002). When you are looking at disorders that affect 1 out of 10, you need to ask how they are defined. As with depression and substance abuse (which are similar in prevalence to ADHD), psychiatric classification can be over-inclusive, failing to distinguish between trait variation and true pathology. ADHD, depression, and alcoholism are all real disorders, yet each lacks a well-defined border that would distinguish it from normality.

Psychologists describe this problem in the terms of the need to separate *traits* from disorders. Although that principle is best established for personality disorders, it could apply to most, if not all, diagnoses in psychiatry (Livesley, 2001). Traits are normal variants that differ from one person to another. They can work for people under some conditions but create problems under other conditions. We might describe traits with a score on a dimension, as we do with blood pressure. You just need to establish a cutoff point at which variations on a dimension are most likely to become pathological. Disorder would be defined by harmful dysfunction (much like a blood pressure of 140/90). Unlike phenomena such as delusions or hallucinations, traits are universal, not symptoms that most people never experience. In the case of ADHD, differences in attention, activity, and impulsivity are all traits that can be functional or dysfunctional. Everything depends on context.

The DSM-IV-TR divides ADHD into three types: one characterized mainly by hyperactivity, one by inattention, and one by a combination of both (American Psychiatric Association, 2000). The overall diagnosis can be established by having either 6 listed features of increased activity or 6 listed features of decreased attention. The Connors rating scale (available on the Internet) is a simple measure with scores on 10 key features of ADHD.[1] The Connors exists in versions for parents and teachers, and in self-report versions for adolescents and adults. It can be used to make a rough and ready diagnosis. But all the Connors really does is to turn DSM criteria into a score.

The largest problem with the DSM definition of ADHD is the inattentive type (Gansler et al., 1998; Nigg & Casey, 2005). In the absence of hyperactivity, problems with inattention alone comprise a set of symptoms that overlap with many other disorders (such as anxiety and depression), making the inattentive type difficult to assess and diagnose (Jensen, Martin, & Cantwell, 1997). Meanwhile, attentiveness is a trait that varies greatly from one individual to another. Some people can maintain attention for hours on end with no difficulty. Others are distractible and have difficulty sustaining the effort to read a book. Moreover, attention may be normal in one context and abnormal in another. For example, few children with ADHD are unable to play games on a computer. Moreover, the clinical problems produced by ADHD can be understood only in a social context—specifically, for example, in a classroom, where young boys are expected to sit down and pay attention. Several generations ago, children who could not cope with that requirement (and there were many) left school at an early age and went out to work. They were not considered abnormal; they were just thought not to be academically inclined. It may be no accident that ADHD was first described in the medical literature about 100 years ago, when child labor was abolished. Once every boy was expected to stay in school until adolescence, one began to see an interaction between traits and social expectations that produced psychopathology.

The third element of ADHD, impulsivity, is even less specific. This trait, when it leads to clinical problems, is also a cardinal feature of *conduct disorder*, a diagnosis that describes serious behavioral disturbances in children (aggression, destruction of property, deceitfulness or theft, and rule violations). ADHD alone may not bring children to clinical attention, and those who are referred may also have a diagnosis of conduct disorder (or a milder form of behavioral disturbance called oppositional defiant disorder) (Maughan, Rowe, Messer, Goodman, & Meltzer, 2004).

Again, "comorbidity" does not mean that children with two diagnoses really have two separate disorders. Conduct disorder (CD) is defined in the DSM-IV-TR by a "repetitive and persistent pattern of behavior in which the basic rights of others or major age-appropriate societal norms or rules are violated" (American Psychiatric Association, 2000). However, the DSM-IV requires that only 3 symptoms (from a list of 15) be present, describing aggression, destruction of property, deceitfulness or theft, and serious violations of rules. Thus, CD is at least as over-inclusive as ADHD itself.

Conduct disorder is more common in boys than in girls; in community surveys it can be found in up to 5% of male children (Moffit, 2001). This high prevalence suggests that CD is still another example of a broadly defined psychiatric diagnosis with unclear boundaries. CD is as much a disease as (but no more a disease than) major depression. Severe cases (those that start early and produce more symptoms) involve a core process of illness that does not usually get better over time (Moffit, 2001). But in children who have only 3 out of 15 symptoms, the diagnosis may not tell us much about outcome.

On the whole, psychiatric categories used for children are even less precise than those that describe adult disorders. This reflects the fact that we know even less about child psychopathology than about mental illness in adults. There is an obvious practical value in diagnosing ADHD, if doing so identifies children who will benefit from Ritalin. Yet not all children meeting the criteria for ADHD respond to Ritalin, and normal children may also concentrate better when they take this drug (Wender, 2000).

Variations in response to treatment raise the question of whether ADHD is a unitary disorder or, like so many other psychiatric diagnoses, a syndrome that could be divided into several diseases. One has to ask whether the widespread use of Ritalin (concentrated in the United States) is always a rational medical prescription, or whether it can be used as a means of controlling uncontrollable behavior, as a simpler alternative to other strategies.

One possible advantage of diagnosing ADHD in children is that it can predict sequelae in adults. Researchers have found that patients with childhood ADHD do not necessarily "grow out of it" but may continue having symptoms as adults (Rutter Kim-Cohen, & Maughan, 2006a; Weiss & Hechtman, 1993). And adults with ADHD may also benefit from stimulant therapy (Weiss & Hechtman, 1993).

In fact, ADHD is now being frequently diagnosed in adults. But given a broad definition and fuzzy boundaries, it is hard to say who has the disorder and who does not. All kinds of people who have trouble concentrating (and even many who have problems with work and relationships) are coming into our clinics and offices asking if they have ADHD. The disorder certainly does exist in adults, but it is a concept that has been used to explain a very wide range of symptoms. It has become a fashionable diagnosis, greatly reinforced by media attention. After hearing about it on television, many patients come to see psychiatrists and family doctors convinced that their problem is ADHD. In my own consultations, this has become one of the most common questions I am asked.

Again, not every problem in attention is the same. Many people have trouble concentrating in some situations but not in others. For example, people who have difficulty maintaining enough attention to schedule and perform a task might be understood as procrastinators. Moreover, problems with attention can be associated with depression, anxiety, or personality disorders. When psychiatrists choose to use broad diagnostic criteria based on a widespread and nonspecific symptomatic picture, they may find that a large portion of the population meets them.

It would help if we had biological markers that could identify who has ADHD and who does not. There have been interesting research findings showing biological abnormalities in some children with the diagnosis. Researchers are looking for genes, but no associations have been found that are specific to ADHD (Thapar, O'Donovan, & Owen, 2005). Although neuroimaging studies point to abnormal patterns of activity, we cannot diagnose ADHD with a brain scan (Doyle et al., 2005). If we could, we might be in a better position to discriminate between those most likely to respond to stimulants and those unlikely to benefit.

In principle, one cannot diagnose the adult form of ADHD without proving that it began in childhood (Weiss & Hechtman, 1993). Yet it is often difficult to be sure. Some children may have never received treatment for their problems. One needs a clear history of dysfunction, such as frequently causing disruptions in the classroom or failing in school. Many of the adult patients I have seen who ask for ADHD treatment have no such history. Often they functioned reasonably well in grade school and high school but began to have problems when they were expected to meet more demanding requirements. Many patients complain of attentional problems at their job, but on inquiry it becomes clear that they are anxious, depressed, substance abusing—or just bored. These problems are not necessarily caused by ADHD. As we saw in the case of depression, patients today are often looking for an explanation (preferably a chemical imbalance) for their problems. Ritalin is another potential quick fix.

In addition, one should keep in mind that a therapeutic response to methylphenidate does not prove that a patient has ADHD. This drug is a stimulant related to amphetamine. It improves attention in everyone, including normal people (Volkow, Wang, Fowler, & Ding, 2005). (In the past, students took amphetamines just before an exam.) Assuming that a drug response affirms a diagnosis is the same kind of mistake we have seen in the diagnosis of mood disorders: Just because patients feel better with an antidepressant does not mean the main problem was depression.

A real category has been used as an explanation for too broad a range of symptoms. As with lithium's use for bipolar disorder, the use of Ritalin for ADHD was a great success. But psychiatric fads can emerge from effective forms of treatment. Practitioners may want to build on success by treating patients with related problems identically. The fact that Ritalin helps children (and some adults) with ADHD has led to using drug prescriptions as easy solutions for a wide range of problems.

The Boundaries of PTSD

PTSD is another problem child, and the intense interest in this disorder is a social phenomenon. No one wants trauma to happen, and we sympathize with its victims. Yet PTSD has become a metaphor for the hope that we can heal all sufferers—or to heal society itself. This is, of course, a tall order.

It has been known throughout human history that traumatic experiences can lead to long-term effects (McNally, 1999). However, the description of a specific medical syndrome associated with trauma appeared only in the 19th century, largely as a result of observations of the effects of combat during the American Civil War. Since then, post-traumatic symptoms have been described after major conflicts (Young, 1995). In World War I, the effects of combat exposure were called "shell shock." In World War II, a similar syndrome was called "combat fatigue." The experiences of psychiatrists working with Vietnam veterans led to the present construct of posttraumatic stress disorder (PTSD).

In recent years, psychiatrists have become increasingly interested in civilian trauma (McNally, 1999). Concerns about the status of women led to greater interest in the impact of rape. Concerns about the effects of crime and violence led to research on the effects of exposure to such events. There has been particular interest in the impact of trauma on children.

DSM-III introduced PTSD as a specific category after Vietnam veterans' groups lobbied for its inclusion. A large number of patients were seeking treatment in Veterans Administration hospitals, and they needed a diagnosis to validate their treatment. However, as documented by the medical anthropologist Allan Young, most patients had problems that did not start in Vietnam (Young, 1995). Many had suffered—including from substance abuse and behavioral problems—before serving in the military, and thus their symptoms could not be explained by trauma alone, even if doing so gave them the right to free therapy.

Psychiatrists, like everyone else, can have strong emotional reactions to trauma histories. In their haste to validate a patient's experience, they may invoke PTSD when patients develop any form of symptoms after a traumatic event. But the definition in DSM-IV-TR is much more specific: Diagnosis requires recurrent intrusive recollections, emotional numbness, and a sensitivity to environmental triggers that resemble the original stressful event (American Psychiatric Association, 2000). Diagnosis is also affected by the time frame: Symptoms lasting less than a month are termed "acute stress reaction," symptoms lasting up to three months are termed acute PTSD, and symptoms lasting more than three months lead to a diagnosis of chronic PTSD. Acute stress reaction is most common, acute PTSD less common, and chronic PTSD less common still (Paris, 2000b).

Posttraumatic stress disorder is one of the few categories in the DSM system that has etiology built into its definition. Yet there are several problems with the idea that PTSD is caused by traumatic experiences (Paris, 2000b). First, how do we define trauma? This word has been overused to the point that almost any negative life event can be called "traumatic." We would be better advised to use this term for events (such as rape or other violent crimes) that are particularly likely to lead to sequelae.

Second, how do we define stress? That term tends to be used to describe a variety of challenges in life. But one's response to the stressfulness of events depends on one's personality. Calling an event too "stressful" tends to imply that it derives from circumstances totally beyond one's control.

Third, most individuals exposed to trauma will not develop symptoms (Yehuda, 1999; Yehuda & McFarlane, 1995). Even the most disastrous life events do not necessarily lead to mental disorder. Most war veterans, even those who have been in the bloodiest of battles, never develop PTSD. Of those exposed to combat, about 25% will present this clinical picture. After non–life-threatening events (such as mild car accidents), rates are even lower. In fact, about 20% of people are exposed to some kind of traumatic event in the course of a year, but the annual prevalence of PTSD in the community is only 1%.

Ultimately, the explanation given to clarify and justify the diagnosis is that people who develop PTSD are more vulnerable than others to stressful events. Long-term sequelae are more likely in those who already have symptoms. In a famous study of Australian firefighters, researchers were able to predict who would develop PTSD by assessing personality traits and by determining past exposure to stressors (McFarlane, 1989). Genes also play a role in shaping vulnerability. In a large sample of twins who served in the Vietnam War, researchers found that *all* the symptoms of PTSD were heritable (True et al., 1993). Vulnerability to this disorder precedes the development of the clinical picture. Thus, PTSD is not *caused* by, but only *triggered* by, traumatic events.

If psychiatrists were to follow the DSM manual carefully, they would not over-diagnose PTSD. But that is not what is happening. The over-diagnosis of this syndrome comes not from algorithms but likely from compassion. Perhaps we are particularly sensitive to these issues (many of us chose this kind of work to help the afflicted). At the same time, we are professionals who are part of a larger culture. Wars and massacres are documented on television, leading to a worldwide moral consciousness that affects us all.

Unlike ADHD, then, the trend to diagnose PTSD is not driven by a wish to expand the application of a successful treatment. Therapy *can* nonetheless often be successful: Many patients respond to CBT, which is probably the most effective treatment (Foa, Rothbaum, & Furr, 2003). In spite of massive marketing, however, the method called eye movement desensitization and reprocessing (EMDR) has produced no better results than have the standard methods that psychologists have been using for years (Devilly & Spence, 1999). And many people recover from PTSD without any therapy all. Forcing people exposed to trauma (as has been sometimes done with children after school shootings) to undergo counseling or "debriefing" tends to make things worse, not better (McNally, 2003).

After 9/11, it was suggested that professional help would be needed for survivors, for families—and even for the millions of people who only witnessed the event. That was an unscientific claim. While those who narrowly escaped with their lives were more likely to develop symptoms, there has been no epidemic of psychological dysfunction among people who watched the events of 9/11 on television (Foa et al., 2005; Lovejoy, Diefenbach, Licht, & Tolin, 2003).

Like ADHD and bipolar disorder, PTSD is a real illness that has become over-diagnosed. The good news is that most people exposed to trauma are resilient, and do not develop PTSD. Those at greatest risk are vulnerable because of preexisting traits and/or exposure to multiple stressful events (Yehuda, 1999; Yehuda & McFarlane, 1995).

Repressed and Recovered Memories

An extreme manifestation of the idea that traumatic events cause mental illness is found in the concept of repressed memories recoverable through psychotherapy. Although psychoanalysis has fallen into decline, the romance of exploring the unconscious mind retains a certain appeal. One of Freud's early concepts was that repressed memories of trauma produce symptoms (Freud, 1958). Although Freud later concluded that many of these incidents were imaginary, the recovery of traumatic memories was a dramatic idea that formed the basis of many Hollywood films, including such hits such as *Ordinary People*. These movies told stories in which remembering traumatic events, under the care of insightful therapists, led to dramatic cures.

In the last 20 years, much attention has been focused on the idea that childhood trauma can cause a phenomenon called dissociation and that patients can suffer from dissociative disorders, such as multiple personalities. A French psychiatrist, Pierre Janet (1901), coined the term *dissociation* more than 100 years ago to describe a state of mind in which different parts of a person become separated. The popularity of this idea was increased when the psychologist Morton Prince (1906) wrote a book describing a patient with multiple personalities. A later book, turned into the Hollywood movie *The Three Faces of Eve* presented the idea to another generation in the 1950s (Thigpen & Cleckley, 1957). More recently, the idea that dissociation into multiple personalities exists and perhaps results from child abuse was popularized by the best-selling 1973 book by Flora Rheta Schreiber, *Sibyl*, which was also later made into a movie.

Although these cases were colorful, they have always been regarded as rare. There is little doubt that they still are. But in the 1980s, one heard the claim that such cases were actually common but hidden from view (Piper & Merskey, 2004a, 2004b). The idea was also promulgated that hypnotizing patients would produce "recovered memories" that explained how symptoms emerged. In cases marked by dissociative symptoms, these memories would usually involve horrific abuse during childhood. Under the influence of these ideas, an epidemic of "cases" spread across North America.

Dissociative disorders are a diagnostic orphan. In the DSM-II, they had been described as a form of "hysterical neurosis." In the DSM-III, with the demise of the terms hysteria and neurosis, dissociative disorders were grouped separately. Separating them inadvertently contributed to legitimizing the diagnosis, so that, for example, textbooks of psychiatry, which follow the DSM system, all have to have a chapter on dissociative disorders. These disorders were diagnosed much more frequently, and patients were treated with psychotherapies designed to uncover repressed memories of trauma. Unfortunately, both diagnosis and treatment were misguided.

Multiple personality (now relabeled in the DSM-IV-TR as "dissociative identity disorder" or DID) is an artifact of bad (or naïve) psychotherapy (American Psychiatric Association, 2000; Piper & Merskey, 2004a, 2004b). Although it remains possible that a few cases occur spontaneously, patients with a high capacity for dissociation can have symptoms reinforced if therapists are overly fascinated with them.

It is now known that Sibyl's psychiatrist (Cornelia Wilbur) largely concocted her "multiple personalities" (Reiber, 2006). Both Wilbur and the novel's author gained fame (and money) from publicizing the case. Yet Sibyl herself told another psychiatrist that she presented multiple personalities only to please Dr. Wilbur. There was never any documentation of the horrific tales of abuse that Sibyl told. Although we can never know for sure, her stories were probably concocted under the influence of therapist suggestion.

Dissociative disorders represent another diagnostic and therapeutic trend that can be understood in a social context. (This group might be considered an "evil twin" of the legitimate category of PTSD.) Interest in dissociation developed at the same time as national concern about child abuse rose to extraordinary proportions. Although such abuse is indeed more common than previously believed, legitimate concern rapidly turned to mass hysteria. One theory for repressed trauma, proposed by the Boston psychiatrist Judith Herman (1992), suggested that children who are badly abused need to forget these experiences. In fact, the failure to remember abuse was sometimes interpreted as proof that such events *must* have happened.

Therapy based on the concept of repressed traumatic events often made use of hypnosis to "recover" memories. But that method is notoriously unreliable, and, in fact, a large body of research has shown that patients who can be hypnotized are likely to be highly suggestible (Herman, 1992). Under hypnosis, they can produce many dramatic stories, including "satanic ritual abuse." No matter: Dissociation mavens claimed that satanic rites were indeed occurring and involved the killing of babies, yet no one ever found the corpses of these supposedly murdered infants. What was happening was that entirely false memories were being produced under the prompting of therapists with strong preconceptions.

The recovered memory epidemic was based on a false psychological theory. Therapists, beginning with Freud, believed that everything that happens in one's life is recorded in the brain. It was thought that memory is a kind of tape recorder (or video recorder) of one's whole life. But that is not true. We do not remember most of what happens to us, and what we do remember is more of a narrative than a recording (McNally, 2003). Memories of the past are rarely factually accurate. We tell old stories in new ways, re-creating and reinterpreting the past in light of the present. Few people can remember childhood experiences with accuracy. Most cannot remember anything before the age of 3. Thus the memories of patients with dissociative disorders (or others subjected to recovered-memory therapy) are mostly fabrications shaped by a desire to please therapists or to explain current problems.

Unfortunately, the concept of repressed memories for trauma led to a rash of unwarranted accusations against families, particularly accusations of childhood incest (Piper & Merskey, 2004a, 2004b; Reiber, 2006). False memories, created and reinforced by therapist suggestion, tend to favor the most dramatic possible events.

Bad therapy practices were destroying lives (and families), but the epidemic was not confined to clinical settings. Lurid charges of sexual abuse were also made against daycare workers, and suggestible children were convinced to testify against them in court. Many innocent workers were convicted, and it took years to secure their release from prison.

Eventually, a reaction set in. A turning point occurred when a California therapist was successfully sued by a father unjustly accused of sexually abusing his daughter (Johnston, 1999). Another came when a psychiatrist at the University of Chicago, who ran a unit for the treatment of dissociative disorders, was sued for millions and lost his license (Grinfeld, 1999). And a mother whose ex-husband had been falsely accused founded the False Memory Foundation to combat these bizarre misuses of therapy.

Yet many of these excesses and outrages were supported, at least to some extent, by institutional psychiatry. Dissociative disorders were never removed from the DSM. Legitimacy for the diagnosis was provided by journals and textbook chapters written by "experts"—usually true believers who multiplied personalities for a living. The former longtime editor of the *American Journal of Psychiatry,* John Nemiah, was a firm supporter of the movement.

Dissociation as a symptom is a real phenomenon. We all have the experience, when driving long distances, of being unable to remember how we got from point A to point B. Some people dissociate under stress—this usually consists of experiencing feelings of unreality; psychiatrists call it "depersonalization." However, there are vast individual differences in the occurrence of such reactions. Again, a symptom does not make a disease.

Everyone loves a drama. Multiple personality provided a wonderful theatrical performance, involving both patients and therapists. It has a story, with a victim (the patient) and a villain (the abuser from the patient's past). This is probably why this concept has more of a future in Hollywood than in a scientific psychiatry.

Personality and Personality Disorders

I have described boundary problems affecting some of the most important diagnoses in psychiatry—major depression, bipolar disorder, and
attention-deficit hyperactivity disorder. But to be fair, my own area of
research and practice—personality disorders—is afflicted by many of
the same problems—fuzzy boundaries between normal variation and
pathology.

Personality disorders are among the most difficult of psychiatry's
problem children: these are patients we are forced to look after, even if
we do not want to. The concept of a personality disorder describes a
patient with chronic emotional and behavioral problems that begin early
in life and go on to affect work and relationships over many years. Thus
this construct goes beyond the presence of specific symptoms. But for
some, the idea is associated with the excesses of the past—one of those
fuzzy ideas promoted by psychoanalysis that only Woody Allen would
take seriously. All the same, psychiatrists often treat these cases with
varying degrees of success.

The DSM-IV-TR places these conditions on Axis II and lists 10
categories of disorder (American Psychiatric Association, 2000). But
there are many problems with the Axis II system. The first is that its
categories do not fit patients very well. One recent study found that about
half of patients meeting the overall criteria for a personality disorder do
not fit into any of the categories (Zimmerman, Rothschild, & Chelminski,
2005). The DSM handles this problem by allowing a diagnosis of "personality disorder, not otherwise specified" (NOS). (An "NOS" category is
an escape route provided by the manual for almost all groupings, including anxiety and depression, when criteria do not fit a case.)

The second problem is that it is almost impossible to determine
where normal traits end and where personality disorders begin. Everyone
has a personality (individual differences in emotion, thought, and behavior). Sometimes our personality works for us and sometimes it does
not. Our friends and intimates can attest to this. At what point does the
failure of these traits become pathological?

This difficulty in separating normal variations in personality from
disorder leads to a third problem: Quite a few of the Axis II categories
lack good evidence for their validity (Livesley, 2001). For example,

obsessive-compulsive personality disorder describes people who are more or less "control freaks." But its high community prevalence (close to 8% in one study) is a warning sign that its criteria are too broad, drawing too many people into the net (Grant et al., 2004).

Only two or three categories listed on Axis II describe valid clinical entities. One of them is antisocial personality disorder (Black, 1999). This diagnosis is a common adult outcome of childhood conduct disorder (one cannot even make the diagnosis without establishing that problems began in childhood). This category describes patients with irresponsible and criminal behavior who are commonly seen in the legal system but who typically do not seek treatment. However, every psychiatrist has experience with these cases, patients who come to our attention only when they are up on charges. (A more severe subgroup of antisocial patients has been described and studied under the diagnostic term "psychopathy" [Hare, 1999].)

The second category that has reasonable validity is borderline personality disorder (BPD) (Gunderson, 2001). This happens to be my special interest, but anyone working in the mental health professions will be familiar with these patients. They come to clinics and emergency rooms, often after repeated overdoses and self-cutting. They experience unstable emotions, with rapid shifts of mood from depression or anxiety to anger. They present with a wide range of impulsive actions—chronic suicidal behavior, self-mutilation, angry outbursts, and substance abuse. Interpersonal relationships are conflictual and unstable. Quite a few BPD patients also experience hallucinations under stress. There is little doubt that these patients suffer from a mental illness.

A third category that has been the subject of research is schizotypal personality disorder (Siever & Davis, 2004). But that diagnosis can be understood as a mild form of schizophrenia that might be better classified within that spectrum (as it is in ICD-10).

Personality disorders are another example of how the loose boundaries of psychiatric diagnosis cause problems. We could put almost anyone with serious relationship problems or work conflicts in this general category. The frequent suggestion that these disorders might be better described by scores on personality traits only reinforces how difficult it is to distinguish life problems from mental disorders.

It may have been an error to place personality disorders on a separate axis from other common mental disorders in the DSM-III. While the intention was to give these problems more attention, the result was the creation of an "Axis II ghetto" that can safely be ignored. The Axis I–Axis II distinction in the DSM system also determines who gets treated and who does not. If a diagnosis is not listed on Axis I, it is not covered. Because BPD is coded on Axis II, many insurance companies will not pay for its treatment. (Meanwhile, insurance has often covered expensive treatments of dissociative disorders because they were placed on Axis I.)

At the same time, continuous efforts have been made to eliminate personality disorders from psychiatry, particularly by mood disorder researchers who, as discussed in the last chapter, describe them all as variants of Axis I disorders because they wish to prescribe medication to treat them. If patients with personality disorders are depressed (as many of them are), their physicians may focus on that one symptom and prescribe antidepressants. But patients with Axis II disorders do *not* respond well to medication, and because current practice encourages psychiatrists to keep trying to get a response, the result is often "polypharmacy," in which patients receive as many as four or five drugs because none of them works well (Zanarini, Frankenburg, Khera, & Bleichmar, 2001).

Including these disorders on a separate axis in the DSM may have been a concession to psychoanalysts who believed they could change personality structure through psychotherapy. And, indeed, this group of disorders remains a domain where talk therapies, including both cognitive and psychodynamic methods, are paramount. As shown by a series of clinical trials, highly impaired patients in the borderline category can benefit from skilled psychotherapy—precisely the modality that most psychiatrists have forgotten how to provide (Paris, 2005b).

Conclusion

Research and treatment using current DSM categories are bound to suffer until the boundary problems with diagnosis are solved. When does inattention become ADHD? When do reactions to stress become PTSD? At what point does personality itself become a disorder? In the absence of biological markers to determine these boundaries, and in the absence of clearly defined conceptual distinctions between normal and abnormal, invalid categories will continue to be classified as real illnesses so long as the DSM system encourages that trend.

TREATMENT

7

Evidence-Based Psychiatry

Medicine as an Art and as a Science

Someone could go to 10 psychiatrists for a problem and get 10 different opinions about what the best treatment would be. This variability is not unique to psychiatry but is a problem for all of medicine. Without agreed-on standards, practice can be more of an art than a science. As a whole, treatment options have long been afflicted by the dominance of clinical opinion, and in many ways, the history of medicine is rather sobering.[1] In the past, physicians worked without any standards for determining whether their treatments worked. Practice depended almost entirely on the accumulation of experience. (That is why bleeding and purging survived for centuries.)

This is not to say that the medicine of the past had no science behind it. Over the past century, practice has benefited greatly from research—to take an obvious example, data show the specific benefit of antibiotics for bacterial infections. In this area, science led to rational practice, in which prescriptions could be based on culturing organisms and determining to which drug various organisms were most sensitive (even if this procedure was not consistently followed). Yet, wherever there was controversy in medicine, it was still settled by opinion.

The first randomized controlled trial (RCT), which examined the effectiveness of streptomycin to treat tuberculosis, was conducted in the 1940s, and RCTs gradually became the gold standard for evidence-based treatment. However, even when new data became available, physicians did not necessarily consider it. For example, studies published in the 1970s with long-term follow-ups, showed that performing "radical" mastectomy to treat breast cancer was no more effective than simply removing a lump of malignant tissue (Fisher et al., 2002). Yet, when these results first came out, many surgeons refused to change their practice, insisting that they could not deny their patients the "benefit" of the more radical procedure.

Today the practice of medicine is much less authoritarian and bound to tradition than it was when I was in medical school. Patients are more likely to be involved in decision making about their care, and they can be almost as current about the results of scientific medicine as their physicians are. Many advances in medicine or results of new research are openly discussed on television and the Internet, and patients react to the information. For example, a few years ago new research raised doubts about the value of hormones to treat the symptoms of menopause and found some danger associated with hormone replacement therapy. Many women stopped taking these drugs as a result. Since that time, recent data suggests that hormone replacement therapy still has a role for some patients, and it is likely that many educated consumers are also aware of this finding (Pitkin et al., 2005).

But despite the vast accumulation of research into disease treatment, some more than a century old, medical practice remains largely an art. There are very few decisions that physicians make that have been definitively examined by research findings, and it is not only in psychiatry that patients get different advice from one doctor than from another.

Why Clinical Experience Alone Is Not Sufficient

Traditionally, doctors' authority has rested on their clinical experience. Even today, silver-haired (and silver-tongued) physicians are held in higher esteem—with patients, colleagues, and the general public. One should not dismiss experience entirely. I would not wish to discount the fact that I have seen 20,000 patients in my lifetime—and may even have learned something from doing so!

Nonetheless, conclusions based on clinical experience suffer from two serious flaws. The first is that patients seen by any particular doctor are not necessarily representative of all people suffering from the same disease. Specialists are referred patients with complex and treatment-resistant symptoms. This population is atypical, and specialists with considerable experience can still draw incorrect conclusions. Practice creates an *availability bias,* in which physicians reach conclusions based on the kind of patients they usually see (Groopman, 2007).

The second flaw is that we all see the world through the lens of preconceptions. If doctors have strong beliefs, they will ask certain questions and interpret the answers to those questions to confirm a previous bias. Nobody wants to be wrong, and it is surprising how rarely people change their minds.

For these reasons, there is no substitute in medicine for data collected systematically and independently of any preconception. Doctors may argue over the interpretation of evidence but must bow to the sovereignty of science. The answer to a difference of opinion in medicine cannot be: "If you had as much experience as I do, you would agree with me." It must be: "Let us collect more data and see whose opinion the new evidence supports."

Yet many physicians insist on the primacy of their own experience. When it comes to drugs, I am continually surprised at how people develop "favorites" based on a narrow range of experience with small groups of unrepresentative patients. When it comes to psychotherapy, passions run even stronger. Some of my colleagues, who "know" that long-term dynamic therapy works, dismiss evidence-based medicine because it fails to confirm their clinical experience. It does not occur to them that their practice is limited to a very few well-selected patients. They also have not considered the possibility that their patients might have done equally well with a briefer course of therapy (or no therapy at all).

I am sometimes tempted to be critical of colleagues who believe what they want to believe—whatever the data show. It helps me to be more tolerant (and humble) to remember what I was like earlier in my career. Deep into the practice of psychotherapy and looking for answers to its many problems, I took the views of various gurus in the field very seriously. I now wonder—what was I thinking? None of the authorities who so impressed me had any interest in science or any data to support what they said. Yet I was attracted to their certainty.

In the same way they are applied to psychotherapy, the principles of science must be applied to the assessment of biological treatments. But psychiatrists who prescribe drugs every day to patients are reluctant to doubt their efficacy. Just as psychoanalysts always had another interpretation in hand, biological psychiatrists always have another drug (or combination of drugs) in reserve. Not every psychiatrist has the time or the inclination to critically review the psychopharmacology literature in depth.

In retrospect, medical school was not an ideal place to learn how to think. I remember my biochemistry professor informing us, with ill-disguised disdain, that we were attending a trade school. At the time, he was right—and in some ways he would still be right today. Medical education has gradually improved, and young physicians are now taught to read journal articles, but doctors, for the most part, do not think like scientists. Physicians are in practice to help patients and do not always stop to consider what is known and what is unknown. Science works by requiring that one form hypotheses and test them by carrying out research.

Mental health professionals with a graduate school education are not always that much better. Original research is expected of all scientists who complete a PhD. But even a PhD is no guarantee of a scientific mindset. Robin Dawes is a clinical psychologist who has published provocative critiques of his own discipline. Dawes (1994) notes that a PhD in clinical psychology, originally designed to produce scientific practitioners, failed to do so. Most dissertations by graduate students aiming to be clinical psychologists never appeared in peer-reviewed scientific publications. Moreover, most psychologists who go on to clinical practice take little account of scientific evidence. Science and clinical work do not readily mix.

Evidence-Based Medicine

Evidence-based medicine (EBM) is a movement within medicine that brings science into clinical practice. It applies empirical, quantitative, and statistical methods to determine whether any or all treatments actually help patients (Evidence-Based Medicine Working Group, 1992).

EBM has had a powerful influence on practice, particularly for the younger generation of physicians who have been trained to believe in it. An influential editorial in the *British Medical Journal* describing this concept has been quoted more than 2,000 times since it was published in 1992 (Sackett, Rosenberg, Gray, Haynes, & Richardson, 1996).

EBM has already led to a dramatic change in the contents of medical journals. High-level publications, such as the *New England Journal of Medicine*, the *Lancet*, and the *Journal of the American Medical Association*, rarely publish case reports. (Since single cases prove little, this is not a great loss.) Nor will editors accept articles (commonly published in the past) describing percentages of success in a series of selected patients. Without a control group, that kind of data is almost worthless.

Again, the gold standard for testing efficacy of any treatment is the randomized controlled trial. This is a generally recognized method for assessing drugs, and all other forms of therapy. In an RCT, effectiveness is determined by assigning patients randomly to different treatments, to placebo, or to no treatment. Measures of outcome are "blind" to the therapy that patients actually receive. If there is a well-established method of treatment, the new one should be compared to the old one. But given the fact that many clinical situations are not that cut and dried, most new therapies need to be compared to placebos.

An EBM perspective also encourages physicians to be conservative and to avoid jumping on bandwagons. It has taught us not to depend on single studies but rather on the weight of evidence drawn from multiple studies. It is surprising how often breakthroughs in clinical research fail to be replicated, an indication of the unfortunate fact that positive results are more likely than negative findings to be published or to reach the public through the media. Despite this circumstance, however, the combining of published results from many clinical trials, a method called "meta-analysis," does provide a quantitative measure of the overall strength of findings. In the EBM world, the most rigorous standards are applied by the "Cochrane reports," a set of literature reviews developed and published by a group of researchers in Oxford, U.K.[2] (Given how conservative Cochrane is, any treatment it supports is quite likely to be effective.)

The results of RCTs have disproved or questioned conventional and popular wisdom in several areas. Recently, research has cast doubt on the usefulness of dietary regimes such as calcium supplements for preventing osteoporosis, high-fiber diets for preventing colon cancer, and multivitamin pills for supporting general health (Alberts et al., 2000; Avenell, Gillespie, Gillespie, & O'Connell, 2005; Bender, 2002). RCTs have also raised questions about the usefulness of some of the most common diagnostic methods in medicine, such as routine mammography (Olsen & Gøtzsche, 2006). Usually, drugs long used by physicians tend to have their efficacy supported by RCTs, but with more precise indications. For example, clinical trials show that statins, prescribed for cardiovascular disease, do not prevent cancer (Dale, Coleman, Henyan, Kluger, & White, 2006).

In psychiatry, RCTs have supported the use of antipsychotic drugs for controlling schizophrenia, lithium for preventing the recurrence of bipolar disorder, and antidepressants for treating mood and anxiety disorders (Baghai, Moller, & Rupprecht, 2006; Emsley & Oosthuizen, 2003; Pollack, 2005; Taylor & Goodwin, 2006). At the same time, there have been a few surprises. For example, antidepressants, although effective for depression, are not as superior to placebo as once thought (Moncrieff, Wessely, & Hardy, 2004). Saint-John's-wort, in spite of its popularity as a "natural" remedy, turned out to be not very effective in treating depression (Linde, Mulrow, Berner, & Egger, 2005). And RCTs failed to show that valproate, a mood stabilizer widely used to treat bipolar disorder, is effective to prevent recurrences (Bowden & Karren, 2006). (Such negative findings are not, however, definitive, because it is very difficult to demonstrate preventive effects in long-term chronic diseases.) The point is that you do not know what a treatment can or cannot do without RCTs.

Practice Guidelines

One consequence of the EBM movement has been the development of practice guidelines for each of the major diagnostic categories that psychiatrists treat. Over the last decade, the American Psychiatric Association has published clinical guidelines for diagnoses of all major psychiatric disorders, which are available on the Internet.[3]

These documents, prepared by noted experts on specific mental disorders, are indeed useful—it is better to have some guidelines than none—but they have important limitations. They can be no better than the limited amount of existing data, little of which meets EBM standards. Under these conditions, experts have to resort to lower standards;

consequently, published guidelines end up containing as much clinical opinion as solid data. Often, even the simplest question turns out to be complex, and many answers remain murky. Moreover, since practice guidelines need to recommend some kind of intervention, they can support treatments whose effectiveness is not confirmed by evidence.

One example of guidelines with insufficient evidence supporting them is the use of "treatment algorithms" in psychopharmacology (Salzman, 2005; Trivedi et al., 1998). These are diagrams that guide psychiatrists to move from one prescription drug to another (or to additional drugs) when patients fail to respond to the first attempt at treatment. These guidelines are attractive but not very scientific. Moreover, algorithms encourage polypharmacy—the practice of prescribing several drugs instead of just one. And polypharmacy has never been tested properly or examined to see if its benefits outweigh the harmful side effects of multiple drugs.

The Limitations of Evidence-Based Practice

Many (if not most) activities of physicians have never been subjected to RCTs. For example, a large proportion of surgical procedures have never been tested in that way. Where RCTs are not practical (or are too expensive), EBM suggests that treatment should follow the best evidence— even if that falls short of an absolute standard. Thus, the absence of solid evidence still leaves lots of room for opinion and clinical experience.

Reasons for the lack of solid data derive from the dearth of trials and the artificiality of the RCT method (Westen, 2006). Because clinical trials are expensive, they remain relatively rare. Moreover, patients who sign up for them may not be representative of real clinical populations. Subjects are often recruited through newspaper advertisements, and real patients are not always willing to be randomized for research. Finally, some of the research studies are limited to patients meeting criteria for one specific DSM diagnosis and exclude those who are "comorbid" for any other. The result is that RCTs end up studying only atypical patients who are less sick than the real, complicated patients who psychiatrists see.

One way of resolving these problems is to loosen the rigid rules for conducting RCTs. An *American Journal of Psychiatry* article by a group from Duke University suggested using "practical clinical trials" instead (March et al., 2005). Using this method, researchers would study patients with "real-world" problems who resemble the people seen in clinical practice, as opposed to studying the rarified populations who sign up for research.

Finally, clinical trials, even when multi-centered (i.e., run in several different clinical settings), can easily be rigged by the pharmaceutical industry. Most of these trials compare new drugs against only placebos, not against established methods of treatment.

Why Evidence-Based Psychiatry
May Not Translate to Practice

Human nature being what it is, practitioners tend to learn just enough to avoid being out of date but not enough to be ahead of the tide of change. Every member of the American Psychiatric Association receives a copy of the *American Journal of Psychiatry* monthly. But this is no guarantee that they will read it. People tend to read not out of curiosity, but to focus on what they think they need. And doctors are highly sensitive to their peers' opinions. Thus, in an academic environment, physicians will read the top journals because everyone else is reading them. In nonacademic environments, such as offices or clinics, where there is no such pressure, journals may seldom be read. Many physicians would rather attend talks or listen to tapes and watch DVDs than read journals. An entire medical-update industry depends on these tools. And there will always be some practitioners who will listen more to a pharmaceutical representative than to a professor.

Physicians are driven more by practicality than by curiosity and doubt. Again, practitioners do not think like scientists. They rely more on the last few patients they have seen than on what they read in journals. They also can sometimes be more impressed by a charismatic presentation than by a research article. They do what they think is right, but they may not necessarily practice according to the principles of EBM. When a psychiatrist prescribes a favorite drug even though the evidence for its value is slim, the choice may be based solely on familiarity with that agent. Physicians practice in a way that makes them comfortable. They are understandably skeptical about basing all decisions on data. A standard riposte goes, "Absence of evidence does not prove evidence of absence"—a clever turn of phrase that has nevertheless been used to justify all kinds of bad practices.

The translation of EBM to practice is also less likely when practitioners are worried about the cost of making a mistake. For example, psychiatrists always worry about suicide. In the emergency room, they are faced with this problem every day. Should patients be hospitalized when they threaten to kill themselves? And should patients be admitted after taking an overdose of pills or cutting their wrists?

I have reviewed the literature pertaining to this question and summarized my conclusions in a book (Paris, 2006a). It turns out that the evidence base for the value of hospitalizing patients when they threaten or attempt suicide is slim or absent. Admission is an expensive option that is not supported by data, and yet nobody wants to do a randomized clinical trial in which one possible outcome is suicide.

Based on existing data, there is little or no evidence that psychiatrists know how to predict suicide—or prevent it. You cannot predict anything from suicidal thoughts because thinking about suicide is so common (seen in about 15% of the population in a lifetime). Nor can suicidality provide accurate predictions about whether people will end their own lives. Although about 3% of people who attempt suicide eventually do kill themselves, we do not know how to distinguish them from the 97% who choose to go on living.

I concluded that patients should be admitted to hospital only for specific treatments for mental disorders but not to prevent them from killing themselves. Expensive resources should not be allocated to treatments in the absence of solid evidence for their value. Yet when I have presented these conclusions to my colleagues, I have met with consistent skepticism and resistance. Even those who agree with me are worried that they might be sued for doing the scientifically correct thing. Psychiatrists, like other physicians, often feel they are working under a threat of litigation. Malpractice suits are sometimes successful, even when science is on the side of the physician. This is another reason that doctors are reluctant to give up making decisions based on clinical experience.

The problem with clinical judgment is that no one knows whether it is right or wrong. Common sense is not good enough. What seems obvious may be shown untrue when examined by science. For example, everyone "knows" that talking about a traumatic experience is helpful. This idea evolved into a method called "debriefing" that is often mandated for victims of school shootings or terror attacks. But research has shown that debriefing actually does more harm than good (McNally, 1999). Stirring up feelings after a traumatic event (without helping people process them) is worse than just allowing people to try to put the experience behind them.

Conclusion

The rise of EBM as a guiding principle for practice reflects a change in ideas about physicians' authority. Doctors used to be expected to know the answers to any and all patient questions, and psychiatrists were particularly guilty of speaking from a position of authority, even on issues far outside their own area of expertise. Contrast that past image with the present reality. Patients now expect to be informed about their treatment and to be a part of the decision process, and physicians, including psychiatrists, can even sit down with their patients in front of the computer and research answers together. Medical practice could become more collaborative in this way, although it does make clinical practice more challenging.

Although the clinical practice guidelines we use now are rather primitive, it is much better to have them than to have none. In the long run, idiosyncratic ways of practicing psychiatry will become less common, and physicians will be more accountable, but that is possible only when there is an agreed standard of therapeutics. Ultimately, EBM brings more doubt than certainty to the physician, but that is a good thing. Doctors know much less than they think they do. To encourage humility, one need only examine what psychiatrists believed 50 years ago.

8

Psychiatric Drugs

Miracles and Limitations

Drugs are an essential part of the practice of psychiatry. Over the course of a lifetime, I have seen medication work real miracles in treating mental illness. I can also remember the "bad old days" when effective drugs were unavailable (or not prescribed).

As an undergraduate psychology student in the late 1950s, I volunteered on weekends at a large state mental hospital. This experience gave me the opportunity to see what patients were like before antipsychotic drugs became available. To describe psychiatric hospitals in those days as "snake pits" would not be inaccurate. Patients sat around for years being quietly (or loudly) psychotic, and psychiatrists could do little other than try to calm them down. The methods used included quiet rooms, cold packs, and sedatives such as barbiturates. The first effective antipsychotic drug for schizophrenia (chlorpromazine) was just being tried (in small doses).

All that is now history. When psychiatrists learned how to use antipsychotics properly, hospitals rapidly emptied: These drugs made it at least possible, if not consistently, for patients to live in the community and to benefit from community-based programs. Whatever the inadequacies we faced with those programs then and still face now, I feel little sense of nostalgia for the past (warehousing of the mentally ill in institutions that in many cases were no better than prisons).

And so, antipsychotics like chlorpromazine represented the first miracle that I witnessed in my career. The second miracle was the introduction of effective antidepressants. Whatever their limitations, these drugs have been a boon to humanity. And the third miracle (described in Chapter 5) occurred when lithium was introduced for the treatment of bipolar disorder.

Thus, I have seen dramatic progress in psychopharmacology over the course of my career. But I have also come to realize that we expect too much from drugs and that we now prescribe them too often, with too little data and without serious thought given to other treatment approaches that may also, or instead, be effective for our patients.

Drugs and Medical Progress

The triumph of medicine has largely depended on advances in drug treatment. Only 100 years ago, doctors had few effective medications to offer patients. Antibiotics were unknown, and infectious diseases killed millions. One of the leading physicians of the time, Sir William Osler, stated that morphine (a mainly palliative agent) was the most useful drug in medicine (Bliss, 2002). A few decades earlier, the American physician Oliver Wendell Holmes had remarked ironically, "If all the drugs that had ever been used for the cure of human ills were gathered together and thrown into the sea it would be ever so much better for humanity and ever so much worse for the fishes" (Holmes, 1972, pp. 306–309).

Within a few years after President Franklin Roosevelt died from a massive stroke in 1945, effective treatments for hypertension began to materialize. So did agents that control coronary artery disease, many forms of cancer, and viral infections. Holmes himself would have been impressed as, by mid-century, wave upon wave of new—and more important, effective—medications arrived to change everything in medicine, saving and extending countless lives and improving their quality.

We owe the pharmaceutical industry a debt of gratitude for producing new drugs for people afflicted by a wide variety of diseases. Yet not all research has come from industry. Scientists and physicians, working outside of industry and in universities, have also played a major role. Moreover, drug companies are less innovative than they claim to be, preferring to market "me-too" drugs that are no better than what is already available rather than take a chance on something entirely new. Recently, physicians and even the general public have come to realize that there are serious problems with the way that the pharmaceutical industry operates—particularly its rigging of clinical trials.

Psychiatry has always lagged behind the rest of medicine in therapeutics (Healy, 1999; Shorter, 1997). We had few good drugs until the 1950s, and we tended to rely heavily on other methods, such as electroconvulsive therapy, in the postwar years. Then a group of researchers in France developed the first antipsychotic agent. As so often happens in medicine, the discovery was an accident. Several variants of antihistamines were being tried for anesthesia, and when one was tried out on psychotic patients, it produced dramatic improvement. The results were so astonishing that psychiatrists of long experience (including the dean of British psychiatry, Sir Aubrey Lewis) at first refused to believe them. After so many false starts, here at last was the breakthrough everyone had been awaiting.

By the time I completed my training in 1972, psychiatrists had a useful armamentarium of drugs, falling into four groups: antipsychotics for schizophrenia, tricyclic antidepressants for depression, lithium for mania, and benzodiazepines for anxiety and insomnia. With these agents, we could help many, if not most, of our sickest patients.

The last few decades have brought further progress, but not the kind of breakthroughs that marked the early days of psychopharmacology.[1] Although many new drugs have entered the market, they are generally variants on what we already had. The most important advances have involved the introduction of new groups of drugs that produce the same results with fewer side effects. Because these newer agents are less toxic, they enhance patients' adherence to a medical regime, and both physicians and patients are more comfortable using them.

One should also keep in mind that we do not know how most of the drugs used for mental disorders work. It is entirely possible, however, that advances in neurosciences may lead to further breakthroughs in pharmacotherapy.

Antipsychotics

Since their first availability in the 1950s, antipsychotic drugs have remained highly effective for the purposes for which they were originally developed. A patient who comes to the emergency room in a state of acute psychosis can be "brought down" in hours and will usually be much improved within a few days. Moreover, antipsychotic drugs prevent relapse. Schizophrenic patients generally need to be on maintenance drugs and are likely to fall ill again if they stop taking them. Unfortunately, that happens all too frequently. Antipsychotic drugs are also used for psychoses associated with mania or depression, and for psychotic symptoms with organic causes.

The positive symptoms of schizophrenia—that is, delusions and hallucinations—generally respond well to drugs. But the negative symptoms—such as "flattening" of emotion (i.e., lack of strong feelings of any kind), illogical thought patterns, and loss of will and motivation—do not respond very well. Although maintenance therapy allows us to keep schizophrenic patients non-psychotic, and out of hospital, many remain chronically ill, and very few return to normal functioning. Psychiatrists await the day when research produces drugs that treat the *disease* of schizophrenia—not just its symptoms. A cure for this terrible illness is still far off.

In addition, the side effects of these agents are considerable. The first-generation antipsychotics, the *typicals,* have more side effects than do the second-generation antipsychotics, the *atypicals.* The first antipsychotic, chlorpromazine, produces excessive sedation and low blood pressure, and all the typicals have serious neurological side effects that resemble symptoms of Parkinson's disease—an extrapyramidal syndrome (EPS) marked by restlessness, abnormal movements, and lack of facial expression. Although psychiatrists can "cover" patients with antiparkinsonian drugs to reduce these side effects, they are difficult to eliminate. In the 1970s and 1980s, the most widely prescribed typical antipsychotic was haloperidol (Haldol). This drug is highly potent in small doses and is still used in the emergency room. However, Haldol is particularly likely to produce EPS.

Most worryingly, antipsychotics have long-term effects on the brain, producing a syndrome called *tardive dyskinesia.* This syndrome is characterized by abnormal movements of the tongue and limbs called "tardive" (slow) because they usually only develop after patients have taken the drug for several years. Moreover, tardive dyskinesia, unlike EPS, gets worse over time, and no drug can cure it once it begins.

One of the reasons for the popularity of atypical antipsychotics is that EPS and, more importantly, tardive dyskinesia seem to be less common with their use. However, no long-term studies using large enough samples have been conducted to determine the frequency of tardive dyskinesia. Moreover, the atypicals can have significant side effects of their own. The first atypical, clozapine, for example, was withdrawn from the market in the 1970s because it can suppress the production of white blood cells (a condition called *agranulocytosis*). Because that dangerous side effect can be minimized by careful blood monitoring, clozapine was brought back in the 1990s when it was found to help patients with the most severe and refractory cases of schizophrenia. It did not cure the illness—cases in which schizophrenia resolves entirely with clozapine are rare—but it was considered something of a breakthrough at the time, even making the cover of *Time* magazine as a miracle cure. Today, clozapine is not widely used in practice because of the need to take extra care in monitoring white cells. Nonetheless, some experts think this drug is underutilized, particularly given evidence suggesting that it reduces the high (about 5%) rate of suicide in schizophrenia (Meltzer et al., 2003).

Clozapine has since been overshadowed by safer atypicals. These drugs—risperidone (Risperdal), olanzapine (Zyprexa), and quetiapine (Seroquel)—are now the most widely used antipsychotics. Many psychiatrists assume that the atypicals are, as a rule, more effective than the typicals. In fact, one wonders whether the idea that the newer drugs were a breakthrough was due to their promotion by industry. A large study led by Jeffrey Liebermann of Columbia University, called the Clinical Antipsychotic Trials of Antipsychotic Effectiveness (CATIE), has dispelled the notion of these agents' superior effectiveness: After comparing them with typical neuroleptics for patients with schizophrenia, CATIE showed that the newer drugs are no better for managing psychotic symptoms than are the older ones. Clinical efficacy is equivalent when the older drugs are combined with antiparkinsonian agents to combat the neurological side effects of typicals (Lieberman et al., 2005). And although it has been claimed that atypicals could be effective against the negative symptoms of schizophrenia, there is hardly any evidence to support that idea.

Among the other problems that the atypicals can often cause is a metabolic syndrome, in which patients develop both obesity and diabetes (Newcomer & Haupt, 2006). Psychiatrists have no way to combat these side effects other than changing back to a typical agent. Atypicals are also much more expensive than typicals.

This brings up a more general point. By and large, physicians prefer to prescribe the latest drug, rather than fall back on "golden oldies." We want to be up to date, and therefore tend to believe what we are told by drug companies. Moreover, younger psychiatrists have little or no experience with the older drugs, so falling back on them when problems develop with the atypicals is not an option they are inclined to consider. Yet the treatment of psychosis has not benefited dramatically from the development of atypicals. With the exception of clozapine, the newer drugs do not do anything that the typicals cannot. Side effect profiles are different but may not be better. The real problem is that none of the antipsychotics, although effective for symptoms, cure diseases. We can only hope that agents that can reverse the process of schizophrenia will eventually replace them. To achieve that goal, psychiatrists will have to understand why and how people develop the illness.

Another issue of concern in contemporary practice is that both typicals and atypicals are used for a variety of symptoms that have little to do with psychosis. Today one sees patients treated with neuroleptics for anxiety or for insomnia. This is a bad practice, since one should not prescribe drugs with so many side effects for relatively minor symptoms, particularly given that antidepressants are less toxic alternatives. The "off-label" use of drugs can, in short, often be both unscientific and dangerous.

Antidepressants

Antidepressants were first developed in the 1950s. They are one of the great success stories of modern psychiatry.

The first group of antidepressants, the tricyclics (named after their chemical structure), were developed in Switzerland and within a few years were being prescribed around the world. Tricyclics are effective drugs, but they have unpleasant side effects (such as dry mouth and trouble urinating). For this reason, neither patients nor physicians ever felt fully comfortable with them. The biggest problem was that you could kill yourself with only a week's supply. Newer drugs have since almost entirely replaced them, even though the older group may still be better for severe depression.

Another group of antidepressants, also developed in the 1950s, are the monoamine oxidase inhibitors (MAOIs). These drugs are effective but are rarely used today because of serious side effects. Patients have to be on a special diet to avoid developing dangerous hypertension.

In the 1980s, the selective serotonin reuptake inhibitors (SSRIs) were introduced. Fluoxetine (Prozac), the first SSRI to be marketed in the United States, was described in a best-selling book by Peter Kramer as a "designer drug" (because it was synthesized by Eli Lilly with a chemical structure specifically intended to change serotonin levels in the brain) (Kramer, 1993).

SSRIs had fewer side effects and were much safer than tricyclics—it is difficult to die from an overdose. Like many other psychiatrists, I found I could treat depressed patients more rapidly, probably because patients are more likely to take them. If one warns patients to endure the initial side effects (particularly nausea), most will accommodate to the drug within a week or two. Family doctors also liked SSRIs and now use them so much that psychiatrists have almost stopped seeing "easy" cases of depression. Today many referrals are of patients who have not responded to SSRIs (or to the newer antidepressants).

Many years after their introduction, SSRIs remain a success story. The National Institute for Clinical Excellence (NICE), a British organization that publishes clinical guidelines, has recommended that the standard treatment for depression should be an SSRI (Middleton, Shaw, & Feder, 2005). The American Psychiatric Association guidelines take a similar position (American Psychiatric Association, 2002).[2]

Meanwhile, since the demand for antidepressants is enormous, many alternative agents have hit the market. After Prozac, a number of newer SSRIs were offered, including paroxetine (Paxil), sertraline (Zoloft), citalopram (Celexa), and several others. There is little evidence that any of these are better than (or much different from) Prozac, although some patients do better on one than another. The choice of an SSRI depends more on side effect profiles than on efficacy, and a problem for all the SSRIs is that they cause loss of sexual function (Fava & Rankin, 2002). Many patients complain of loss of interest in sex and/or inability to ejaculate or have an orgasm. Notwithstanding that being depressed also does not make people feel sexual, some patients refuse to take SSRIs because of this side effect.

Since the 1990s, several more non-SSRI antidepressants have been introduced. For example, venlaflaxine (Effexor) has been marketed as an improvement on SSRIs. The manufacturer has had some success in convincing physicians to use this drug as a first-line agent. Advertisements emphasize that venlaflaxine works on multiple sites in the brain (it increases levels of both norepinephrine and serotonin). However, it is not clear what that means or whether the drug is actually better for patients. Another selling point has been that venlaflaxine is less likely to produce sexual side effects, but the evidence behind this claim is also slim. Finally, some studies of venlaflaxine have proposed that it produces more remissions of depression than SSRIs do, but that research was almost entirely paid for by the manufacturer (Roseboom & Kalin, 2000).

Claims of superiority have also been made for other non-SSRIs, such as mirtazapine (Remeron) and buproprion (Wellbutrin), both of which fall into different chemical groups. But there is little reason to believe that these newer drugs are any more effective than SSRIs for depression (Montejo, Llorca, Izquierdo, & Rico-Villademoros, 2001; Shelton, 2004). This is why guidelines for the treatment of depression still recommend (sensibly) that SSRIs be the first choice for most patients, with other agents as backups.

The larger problem is that many depressed patients do not respond, or do not fully respond, to drug treatment of any kind. Antidepressants are less superior to placebo than previously thought (Moncrieff, Wessely, & Hardy, 2004). About 40% of patients get better from depression on their own. At most, half fully recover (go into remission) when treated with antidepressants. And we have no way of predicting which patients are likely to respond to these drugs or which patients do not need them.

The large-scale Sequenced Treatment Alternatives to Relieve Depression (STAR*D), a study funded by the National Institute for Mental Health (NIMH), has produced the most definitive findings about the effectiveness of antidepressants (Trivedi et al., 2006). It showed that the majority of depressed patients experience some degree of symptomatic relief on medication but that about half remain somewhat depressed, even after treatment. About a third of patients may see no benefit at all. Psychiatrists and their patients want to see full recovery, but drug treatment alone does not always deliver that.

When patients fail to get better, one can try a different antidepressant or add another drug (such as lithium or thyroxin). Although these options are indeed used, they have only recently been tested systematically—the main goal of the STAR*D study. That study was designed to determine whether *augmentation* (adding a second antidepressant) or *switching* (to another drug) increases the remission rate in depression.

The findings of the study showed that some patients (20–30%) do benefit from switching or augmentation. So this is an idea worth trying. All the same, there was no further benefit from switching more than once, a point that argues against the practice of trying patients on four or five different antidepressants. The more serious problem that the study identified was that only half of all patients recovered using any drug or combination. Initial prescriptions, followed by augmentation and switching, moved one out of three treatment-resistant cases into remission. In an editorial accompanying this report, David Rubinow of the University of North Carolina noted that many of these patients developed chronic depression (Rubinow, 2004, p. 808).

In a review of this subject, Michael Thase (2004) of the University of Pittsburgh commented, "The fundamental question concerning 'to augment or to switch' is not answerable with available data." Moreover, the Star*D study failed to examine all options. As Thase noted, "The best-documented treatments (i.e., lithium augmentation, switching to a monoamine oxidase inhibitor, and electroconvulsive therapy) are among the least utilized." It has also been pointed out that after 40 years, it has never been shown that any of the other antidepressants are better than a tricyclic (Barbui & Hotopf, 2001).

As it stands, the practice of treating every depression with drugs and of trying more than one agent is questionable. Although antidepressants often work, their efficacy has been exaggerated. Pharmacological options of greater complexity are sometimes effective but do not necessarily work better.

For this reason, augmentation and switching should not be routine procedures, and patients should be informed at the very beginning of treatment that antidepressants may or may not work. Unfortunately, psychiatrists who believe (and convince their patients) that success is just a matter of finding the "right" drug may tell patients they are almost guaranteed to recover—raising expectations that cannot be met or setting up a beneficial, if short-lived, placebo effect. I have seen many patients go through augmentation and switching over months or years without obvious benefit, yet they (and their psychiatrists) keep coming back for more. Again, we need to identify which patients are most likely to remit with antidepressants and to separate them from those who are least likely to benefit.

The Star*D study also investigated non-pharmacological treatments for depression, and its results concerning cognitive therapy have been published (Thase et al., 2007). They show that some patients who do not respond to drugs do better when psychotherapy is added. However, the results were not definitive because many patients (already committed to medical treatment) declined to enter CBT.

Another option is not to prescribe antidepressants at all on the first visit. Some patients improve without them, particularly after a systematic and empathic evaluation. And if they are not better a week later, little is lost by delay (because, in any case, these drugs tend to work slowly). A related problem is that once a patient is on medication, one does not know whether improvement represents a placebo response. Finally, once a drug is started, even if it is not obviously working, physicians can be reluctant to discontinue it and consider other options.

Ultimately, the problem with the uncertain efficacy of antidepressants derives from the fuzzy concept of depression itself (see Chapter 5) and its frequent association with other conditions. Patients with depression do often meet criteria for other psychiatric diagnoses, and in particular, those who have substance abuse and personality disorders do not respond as well to antidepressants (Kocsis, 2003; Newton-Howes, Tyrer, & Johnson, 2006; Nunes & Levin, 2004; Torrens, Fonseca, Mateu, & Farre, 2005). Results in milder chronic depressions (*dysthymia*) are also less predictable (Kocsis, 2003; Newton-Howes, Tyrer, & Johnson, 2006; Nunes & Levin, 2004; Torrens, Fonseca, Mateu, & Farre, 2005). Antidepressants tend to work best in patients who become depressed after having been well and who do not have chronic conditions associated with long-term dysfunction. In addition, many patients have stressful life circumstances—living in poverty or in a difficult family situation—that make them depressed. If nothing is done to improve these circumstances, antidepressants will not be very effective. Drugs work best in those who have fewer reasons to be depressed.

It might be possible in the future to identify, through genetic or biological markers, those patients who are most likely to respond to specific drugs. But psychiatrists will always need to pay attention to who the patient is and to what that patient's story or context is—as opposed to blindly trying to medically regulate a depressed mood.

We also need to consider treatment options besides prescribing antidepressants. For melancholia, electro-convulsive therapy is an effective option that works rapidly. In a classic large-scale study carried out in the 1980s (supported by NIMH), psychotherapy (cognitive or interpersonal) was as effective as antidepressants for all but the most severe cases (Elkin, Shea, Watkins, & Imber, 1989). This finding has been supported by other research (Klerman, DiMascio, Weissman, Prusoff, & Paykel, 1974). Yet, as we have seen, psychiatrists have either not taken into account or do not know the evidence that depressed patients benefit from psychotherapy. Another problem is that talk therapy is less readily available than medication and usually costs more. Nonetheless, at their assessment and before being given a prescription, patients should be informed that psychotherapy is an option. Patients should also be told that evidence shows they are more likely to recover if they receive both drugs and therapy.

In short, depression is more difficult to treat than we think, and it is often a chronic condition. Clinical trials, whether of drugs or talk therapy, need to examine whether patients achieve remission, not just whether they feel somewhat better (Casacalenda, Perry, & Looper, 2002).

Still, for all their questionable overusage, antidepressants remain an essential component of the prescribing physician's treatment approach to depression. Indeed, they are also used to good effect for diagnoses besides depression (Casacalenda & Boulanger, 1998). Patients with anxiety disorders, including panic attacks, and a broader disorder called "generalized anxiety disorder," respond to these drugs, as do patients with obsessive-compulsive disorder. Antidepressants can also suppress symptoms of impulsive disorders, such as bulimia. Even in personality disorders, where their effects are less dramatic, they can often "take the edge off."

In other words, antidepressants have more than one use in therapy, and for that reason, seem to have a misleading name. In some ways they could be thought of as the aspirin of psychiatry: No matter what hurts, it is better to have less pain, and antidepressants can do for many people's psychic pain what aspirin (or other analgesics) can do for many people's physical pain. This comparison is by no means a put-down: Aspirin remains a very effective drug in medical practice and is still used to prevent strokes and coronary artery disease. But its effects are not disease-specific. Similarly, antidepressants are key tools, but their effects are not specific to depression.

In summary, there are limitations to antidepressants: They are often only partially effective and are sometimes not effective at all. We also do not know precisely how they work and why it can sometimes take a few weeks for them to change the brain. We may develop much better drugs in the future. In the meantime, the evidence suggests that psychiatrists should be offering patients a choice among antidepressants, psychotherapy, or both.

Mood Stabilizers

As discussed earlier in this book, the acute manic episodes that patients with bipolar disorder experience can be controlled with antipsychotic drugs. Yet, in contrast to schizophrenia, these agents do not prevent recurrences. That is why lithium was such a breakthrough in the treatment of mania. But lithium is also a drug with serious side effects: Patients can suffer from excessive thirst, develop swelling in the thyroid gland, or develop mild kidney damage.

As long as lithium was the only agent for the treatment of bipolar disorder, patients had to put up with these side effects. And doing so might still be worth it. Even today, the evidence proves that lithium prevents recurrences of mania better than any other drug does (Ghaemi, Soldani, & Hsu, 2003). Research has also suggested that lithium therapy lowers the rate of suicide in bipolar patients (Goodwin et al., 2003). When those with severe depression fail to respond to antidepressants, lithium is the most effective agent that one can add to the treatment (Thase, 2004). This drug remains an essential part of the psychiatric armamentarium.

Today, alternative mood stabilizers, most of which were originally developed as anticonvulsants, tend to be used instead of lithium because they have fewer serious side effects. Even so, the first such agent to be introduced, carbamazepine, was not popular because it reduces the white blood cell count and requires careful monitoring.

Valproate (Depakote or Epival) is the most widely prescribed drug for bipolar disorder. Because it is much less toxic than lithium, it is a useful alternative for many patients. What has not been shown, though, is whether valproate works as well to prevent recurrences. There are also several newer mood stabilizers: topiramate (Topamax), gabapentin (Neurontin), and lamotrigine (Lamictal). But these agents, unlike lithium, have not been shown to be as effective against recurrences of bipolar illness, or against suicide. If a patient has bipolar I disorder (the classical type), lithium is probably the best first choice, with other drugs as backups for patients who cannot tolerate lithium's toxicity.

The success of mood stabilizers in bipolar disorder led to their use for other purposes. Chapter 5 critiqued the theory that a large number of diagnoses in psychiatry are "really" forms of bipolarity and can, therefore, benefit from treatment with the same drugs. This backward reasoning has done damage to patients. The fact that aspirin helps people with a wide range of illnesses does not prove that all such patients have the same disease—or that they suffer from an aspirin deficiency.

A more general concept is that mental illnesses might be classified by applying "pharmacological dissection," that is, by noting differential responses to drugs. This creative idea was proposed many years ago by the Columbia University psychiatrist Donald Klein, who concluded that panic disorder was a separate diagnosis because it had a specific response to medication (Klein, 1987).

However, most drugs in psychiatry work for a wide range of symptoms. Mood stabilizers, like antidepressants and antipsychotics, calm people down, irrespective of cause. Unfortunately, because the symptoms of mood instability are seen in so many other conditions in psychiatry (e.g., substance abuse and personality disorders), a large number of patients are receiving these agents in spite of evidence that they yield only minimal benefit.

Anti-Anxiety Drugs

The main agents physicians prescribe for anxiety are the benzodiazepines (called "benzos" for short). These drugs include diazepam (Valium), lorazepam (Ativan), and clonazepam (Klonopin or Rivotril). Although all these agents reduce anxiety (and help people sleep), the longer patients take them, the less effective they are. Like alcohol, they induce tolerance (a need for higher doses), and some patients become physically addicted (Stevens & Pollack, 2005). It is therefore a good idea to use benzodiazepines only for a short time. There are also long-acting "benzos" (such as clonazepam) that produce fewer problems with tolerance.

Benzodiazepines are often prescribed by family doctors, but psychiatrists also prescribe them regularly for anxiety and insomnia, whatever their patients' diagnosis. In fact, these drugs are vastly overused, insofar as anxiety and insomnia do not always respond to them. When that happens, the benzodiazepines can be replaced with antidepressants, which continue to work over time and do not cause addiction.

The Limitations of Psychiatric Drugs

Within one generation, advances in drug therapy changed the way psychiatrists practice, and then the rate of progress slowed down. We would be shocked if internists treated every disease with an arsenal as limited as the one we have. In fact, most of the choices that psychiatrists have when they write prescriptions lie between standard agents and copycat drugs that the pharmaceutical industry is promoting to break into a lucrative market. Although some newer drugs are safer, we are still working with the same basic groups we had 30 years ago. Unfortunately, there is no reason to believe that psychiatrists are that much better at treating mental illness than they were then. Moreover, they are prescribing drugs far beyond what the evidence shows are their indications.

For as long as I can remember, our specialty has gone from one extreme to another. Forty years ago, psychiatrists who "believed" in psychotherapy made insufficient use of drugs—to the detriment of their patients. Today drugs are almost the only treatment psychiatrists offer, and they are prescribed routinely. A balanced view would at least try to differentiate between situations where drugs are essential and where they are optional (or unnecessary).

Prescribing drugs runs parallel to reducing the use of psychotherapy, even though the evidence for the effectiveness of talk therapies in milder or moderate forms of depression is just as strong as it is for the effectiveness of medications. When drugs and brief therapies are compared directly, they work equally well for many people. Moreover, a combination of medication and therapy has been shown to be more effective than either treatment alone. Drugs are most necessary when patients suffer from illnesses of greater severity.

We have known for many years that patients with depression are more likely to recover when offered a combination of drugs and psychotherapy (as opposed to either alone) (Klerman et al., 1974). Prescribing both forms of treatment "covers" both patients who mainly respond to medication and those who respond best to talk therapy. At the same time, the two modes of treatment have synergistic effects, targeting different aspects of depression (e.g., physical symptoms versus depressed thinking).

Drugs are most necessary when patients suffer from illnesses that are more severe. Yet research has shown that even in the treatment of those illnesses that absolutely require drugs (schizophrenia and bipolar disorder), cognitive-behavioral therapy offers added value for rehabilitation (see Chapter 9). Nevertheless, very few patients with psychotic disorders receive this or any other psychotherapy—the human resources are almost always lacking.

Given the scientific evidence, why do so many patients receive *only* drugs? Why do psychiatrists not even *think* of prescribing psychotherapy when patients fail to respond to medication or when the addition of psychotherapy is known to effectively augment a medical regimen?

These problems relate to issues raised in the earlier chapters of this book. At least part of the answer lies in reductionist thinking about mental illness—and in the field's hope that psychiatry, like other areas of medicine, will define specific diseases with unique responses to treatment, much as infections respond to specific antibiotics. Thus, the belief that, say, major depression is a unique disease supports the practice of giving antidepressants to any patient who meets criteria for that disorder—in spite of the evidence discussed above that results are not consistent.

Another part of the answer lies in the limitations of time and money, and in the human resources problem. It takes only a few minutes to write a prescription (although making sure the patient actually fills it and takes it might require a little more time), whereas psychotherapy, even the evidence-based brief therapies, take more time, a very scarce resource for psychiatrists and patients.

Most of all, it is the pharmaceutical industry that drives the practice of over-prescription. In their advertising, the companies always claim greater efficacy for newer drugs, pitching them to physicians who worry about being out of date. Yet many drugs whose patents have long since expired are excellent if used properly (for example, typical neuroleptics and tricyclic antidepressants).

Treatment Resistance and Treatment Algorithms

The failure of some patients to respond to drug therapy has sometimes been called "treatment-resistance" (Keller, 2005). This usually refers to a scenario in which depression is specifically resistant to standard drug treatment. The response to this scenario by many psychiatrists is not to reassess the nature of the patient's depression but to prescribe yet more drugs. Thus, when patients fail to respond to an older drug, they receive a prescription for a newer one. Or, succumbing to pressure from the pharmaceutical industry, the psychiatrist may prescribe the newer agent first (Angell, 2005; Avorn, 2004). New drugs are being aggressively marketed even though they are no better than what we already have. A cynic might say that the drug companies need to develop new antidepressants every 10 years or so because the patents on the old ones run out.

The failure of depression to respond routinely to antidepressants reflects our overly broad definition of the disorder. As discussed in Chapter 5, patients falling within the category are a very mixed bag, including "classical" cases of melancholic depression, in addition to cases in which people are unhappy and miserable because of life circumstances and/or a disordered personality. Because antidepressants are being prescribed for a mixed category of illness, it is not that surprising that the results are mixed. "Garden-variety" depression is probably not the same illness as melancholia (in which patients feel either agitated or sluggish and cannot function at all).

Another explanation for treatment resistance is "comorbidity" (First, 2005). The implication is that drugs have not worked because the patient has more than one disease. Yet, as discussed in Chapter 3, the DSM system yields multiple diagnoses in many (if not most) patients. What comorbidity should actually tell us is that the clinical problem is more complicated and that one may not be looking at a "classical" form of illness. Somewhere between a quarter and a half of depressed patients suffer from comorbid personality disorders (Zimmerman, Rothschild, & Chelminski, 2005). Again, this is a population with serious and long-term life problems in work and relationships that both cause and impede recovery from depression and who do not respond as well to antidepressants (Newton-Jones, Tyrer, & Johnson, 2006).

All these considerations go by the boards in the endless search for the "right" medication. It is worth trying a second drug if the first fails. But as described in Chapter 7, psychiatrists have been encouraged to follow *treatment algorithms*—procedures that describe sequences of treatment options to be followed when first attempts fail (Fawcett, Stein, & Jobson, 1999). These algorithms are found in many of the guidelines published and endorsed by the American Psychiatric Association. However, research into their efficacy is very much in its early stages. As we have seen from the STAR*D study, multiple options are definitely worth considering but they are not *necessarily* useful. Reading Cochrane reports would no doubt support a conclusion that algorithms lack high-quality evidence to be practical guides.

Polypharmacy

Nevertheless, treatment algorithms have become an entrenched part of clinical practice, and because they describe treatment of a variety of different symptoms in patients, they encourage *polypharmacy*. Some patients with a wide range of symptoms can end up on as many as four or five drugs (Zanarini, Frankenburg, Khera, & Bleichmar, 2001).

More than 100 years ago, William Osler (1898) raised questions about these practices. Even then, there was a tendency to manage every symptom in medical patients with a different prescription. (Although drugs are usually more specific to symptoms than to illnesses, that only reflects the fact that diagnoses are not well defined.) As we have seen, many pharmacological agents have overlapping effects. And as the STAR*D study showed, adding medication runs up against a law of diminishing returns. Moreover, each medication has its own side effects, some of which can be cumulative. What is most concerning about polypharmacy is the almost complete lack of clinical trials on the effects of drug combinations. Even if every individual drug prescribed were well supported by data, we would not be able to predict what happens when we give them in combination.

Polypharmacy, like other practices discussed in this chapter, can sometimes reflect physician frustration. If one drug does not work, we try another. But since we may be reluctant to remove the first agent, we just add the second one. And the same applies to the third, the fourth, and so on.

Psychopharmacology in Children and Adolescents

At one time, a psychoanalytic perspective dominated child psychiatry—even more than it did for adults. Today the change to a biological paradigm has spread across all age groups. Drug treatment for children has become the norm. This is not to say that pharmacology for children need be wrong—as discussed in Chapter 6, Ritalin has been documented to be effective in well-diagnosed cases of ADHD. But children present with many other diagnoses and often with a multitude—a level of "comorbidity"—that reflects our inability to categorize their problems. Moreover, adult patients can at least decide whether or not they wish to take drugs for mental disorders; children cannot.

A recent survey found that prescriptions of antipsychotic drugs for children and adolescents have increased by a factor of five over the last decade or so (Olfson et al., 2006). This reflects changes in psychiatry as a whole, in addition to the effects of some of the diagnostic fads described in Chapters 4, 5, and 6. For example, if children with behavioral disturbances are diagnosed with bipolar disorder, they will receive mood stabilizers (and sometimes antipsychotics). In fact, many of the children in the survey were receiving several psychiatric drugs from different groups. The rationale for these multiple prescriptions in children has by no means been established, and no one knows the long-term effects of such regimes.

There is nothing wrong with prescribing drugs when the diagnosis is right and the evidence base is strong. But recent trends suggest child psychiatrists are becoming overly attached to pharmacological tools. No one has properly studied these practices or shown that they do more good than harm. At the same time, child psychiatry may not be making adequate use of advances in psychotherapy, such as the widely researched method of parent-effectiveness training (Kazdin, 1996).

Psychiatry and the Pharmaceutical Industry

One observer, noting the growth of pharmaceutical treatment for both adults and children, has described it as "irrational exuberance" (Rosenheck, 2005). But one cannot understand the way psychiatric drugs are prescribed (and over-prescribed) without considering the influence of the pharmaceutical industry. This is a multibillion-dollar international business that uses its power to influence physicians—and legislators (Angell, 2005; Avorn, 2004).

"Big pharma" spends a small amount of its profits on research but much more on marketing. Representatives of the companies may regularly visit every psychiatrist (and family doctor) in their offices to peddle their wares. And they often come bearing gifts. There are also more subtle ways of buying influence. The pharmaceutical industry gains influence with academic faculty and psychiatric residents by sponsoring their educational activities. This does little harm if the industry provides "unrestricted" grants (money that supports travel for speakers chosen by a university or a hospital). However, many companies sponsor speakers of their own choosing who are paid to support a product. Where these practices are accepted, the pharmaceutical representatives become virtual members of the academic family, ensuring that conferences are held at the best restaurants and that even small seminars offer everyone a free lunch.

Anyone who has ever attended the annual meeting of the American Psychiatric Association (APA) can attest to the overwhelming presence of the pharmaceutical industry there. Drug companies turn APA into a kind of trade fair, with booths handing out all kinds of goodies. Every year I see professionals walking out of the industry section of every conference laden down with gifts, courtesy of Big Pharma. As one of my colleagues asked rhetorically, are psychiatrists so poor that they have to accept pens from industry? It is also possible to attend APA without paying for a single meal.

These practices are marginal but not strictly unethical. In contrast, it is clearly unethical for companies to pay for psychiatrists to attend meetings. There are rules against physicians accepting travel fare or hotel costs from industry. Unfortunately, these guidelines are not always enforced or followed. One way the companies get around rules is to pay psychiatrists as "consultants." Physicians who accept this role get to travel in luxury to vacation spots without having to give anything in return. There is evidence that these "gifts" affects prescribing practices (Wazana, 2000).

Yet most physicians do not believe they are influenced by the pharmaceutical industry. In their opinion, it is not really a problem to accept gifts if doing so does not really influence one's decision as to whether or not any specific drug is prescribed. This view is naïve, and industry has a rather different opinion. Based on marketing research, they *know* that gifts purchase enough goodwill to sell drugs. They also know which doctors are generating sales for their products.

An even more troubling problem is the way that drug companies have dominated clinical trials. Unfortunately, governmental agencies have been less interested in sponsoring these studies. One hardly needs to mention the conflict of interest here—billions of dollars can be at stake. For this reason, the results of trials have sometimes been rigged, by making sure the sample includes patients most likely to respond, by comparing a drug with a placebo rather than with an established agent, or by actually suppressing negative results. The outcry in the media about all these practices has led to new regulations requiring that all trials be preregistered with a central governmental body.

To compound the problem, physicians serving on the Food and Drug Administration, the very body that determines whether or not new agents can be marketed, are often in the pay of industry. Until recently (when the practice was banned), even researchers at NIMH were allowed to take industry money.

Last, but not least, the pharmaceutical industry has exerted a degree of influence on the way psychiatrists classify mental illness. The industry has no direct input into the DSM process, but many of the experts involved in writing the manual are on their payroll (because you can hardly find an expert who does not take industry money).

Influence on diagnostic practices makes a difference. When drugs are indicated for specific diagnoses, companies want psychiatrists to make such diagnoses as often as possible. By sponsoring conferences focusing on a specific diagnostic entity associated with a drug therapy, they encourage psychiatrists to see psychopathology in a certain way and to have the "right" response when considering alternative methods of treatment.

All this might seem to draw a malignant picture of "Big Pharma." But whereas the priority of physicians is patient care, pharmaceutical companies are a business, and their goal is profit. The companies are just doing their job, and it is up to physicians to refuse to be influenced by them.

Whereas some of my colleagues want nothing to do with industry, I try to take a more balanced view. When I was a department chair, I had no problem taking their money to run scientific conferences with "unrestricted" support (i.e., they pay, but we choose the speakers and the topics). But I did not accept industry's own paid speakers. Similarly, as a journal editor, I have no problem accepting advertisements, without which no scientific journal would ever be published. On the other hand, I have been careful about publishing clinical trials sponsored by industry.

Money can corrupt, and the fantastic profits of the pharmaceutical industry have helped corrupt areas of psychiatry. We would not be prescribing so many drugs if it were not for the constant pressure and influence coming from drug companies. Anyone who wants to understand this problem in depth would be well advised to read two recent books: one by Marcia Angell, former editor of the *New England Journal of Medicine,* and one by Jerry Avorn, a Harvard researcher in pharmacoeconomics (Angell, 2005; Avorn, 2004).

The most egregious abuse by the pharmaceutical industry is direct marketing to consumers. This type of advertising, banned in the past, has now become ubiquitous. Pharma's ads encourage patients to talk to their physicians about how they feel and implicitly suggest that they ask for (or even demand) a specific product. Nothing could be more undermining to the practice of medicine.

Of course, physicians do not *have* to be guided by promotional material. Yet, by and large, drug companies have been successful in getting psychiatrists (and family doctors) to do their bidding. Although nothing forces us to prescribe their products, marketing strategies work. And the industry knows it.

In summary, the pharmaceutical industry has convinced psychiatrists to practice in ways that are not in the best interest of patients and that add unnecessarily to the cost of mental health services. For example, while atypical neuroleptics are not necessarily better than typicals, they are routinely prescribed—at 10 times the cost. The same applies to SSRIs, which, although safer, are no more effective against depression than tricyclics that cost almost nothing. (Although tricyclics must be used with caution, they are still useful drugs, particularly for severe depression.) Moreover, psychiatrists have been convinced to try the newest and most expensive antidepressants, in addition to drug combinations, in patients who do not respond well to medication at all. Needless to say, drug companies never encourage psychiatrists to offer psychotherapy to patients.

Conclusion

Drugs are an essential part of psychiatric practice, particularly for patients with severe mental illness. Their effects vary greatly—they can be miraculous or useless but are most often helpful without curing illness. Certainly we need better, safer drugs with fewer adverse effects, and to that end, we should advocate for, encourage, and support the pharmaceutical industry's efforts to develop such agents and to do so based on rigorous, unbiased scientific research. We should also offer patients other kinds of treatment that are non-biological in nature and have been proven effective. The reality, though, is that psychiatrists rely on medication more and more, to the exclusion of any other treatment approach, and it is a tendency that can be understood in many ways. At the very least, it is based not on solid scientific data but on other factors that have little to do with science. The boom in drug prescriptions since the early 1990s for psychological problems can be seen as a kind of "stock market bubble" (Rosenheck, 2005). It is a story of which psychiatrists have little to be proud, with some of us fooled by industry hype or bought out by the industry, and with our patients losing the most.

9

Talk Therapies

The Need for a Unified Method

R esearch shows that psychotherapy is a form of treatment that patients need but do not always receive. Research also shows that no single method of psychotherapy has a monopoly on effectiveness (see Chapter 2), suggesting that the method should not be labeled according to different "schools of thought" but instead should be considered one, integrated discipline. How much time should psychiatrists spend practicing this discipline? And what ideally would its integrated form be? Let us focus on a few possibilities, first by revisiting, for the sake of contrast, a talk therapy that once was the very definition of the term.

The State of Psychoanalysis

Even now, when most laypeople think of psychotherapy, the model that comes to mind is psychoanalysis. Although the method has fallen into decline, it retains residual authority. Psychoanalysis was a broad and ambitious theory that attempted to explain normal human behavior and the origins of mental disorders.[1] Its fall from grace greatly contributed to the current lack of interest among psychiatrists in all forms of psychotherapy.

To avoid throwing out the baby with the bathwater, however, we need to understand why psychoanalysis failed.

Psychoanalysis dominated psychiatry at a time when it faced no credible competition from other psychotherapies. Fifty years ago, at least in the United States, Freud's ideas permeated university departments. This was a time when medicine and psychiatry were less scientific and when dogma and clinical experience were more important than data. When so little was known about mental illness, psychoanalysis filled a niche.

When I trained in psychiatry, its academic leaders often had analytic training. Residents studying psychiatry in leading university departments were expected to learn Freudian theory. The largest residency program in U.S. psychiatry was located at the Menninger Clinic in Kansas, an institution deeply committed to the psychoanalytic movement.

Fantastic as it seems in retrospect, only a few questioned its methods or its effectiveness. Even psychiatrists not formally trained in analysis saw the world through its perspective. Many young practitioners expected to spend their career seeing patients several times a week for years. Anything less was considered superficial and unhelpful. The public perception, which equated psychiatry and psychoanalysis, was not that far off the mark.

The problem was that analysts, in spite of their claims to be "scientific," were untrained in research methods and never published systematic or quantitative reports. The psychoanalytic enterprise rested on hypotheses that were never tested—it was based on unquantifiable "data" such as free associations and dreams. Moreover, what analysts heard from their patients was shaped by their own preconceptions. And what patients said was based on what they thought their analysts wanted to hear. As science, this approach can only be described as hopeless.

The psychoanalytic movement is now more than 100 years old. For psychiatrists to accept the authority of Sigmund Freud today would be like internists now relying on treatments recommended by Freud's contemporary, William Osler. However, Osler was a pioneer of evidence-based medicine, whereas Freud never conducted (or encouraged others to conduct) research; consequently, his method never became anything resembling a science. Analysts never tested their hypotheses against data, and few of them actually understood how science works. Instead, they told stories about human behavior and treated them as truth. These narratives were sometimes plausible. Sometimes they were simply bizarre. But even stories can be measured and tested.

Psychoanalysis also suffered from intellectual isolation, having little contact with other disciplines. Freud had responded to rejection by European academic psychiatry by creating independent "institutes" devoted to teaching his ideas and his method. Psychoanalysis came to resemble a religion, and training to be an analyst was more like becoming a priest than like becoming a doctor. As with so many other religions, the movement became intolerant, rooted in dogma, and divided by schisms. Held back by rigidity and conservatism, creative thinkers were forced out of the movement. Psychoanalysis, more of a cult than a branch of science, ended up having stronger links with the humanities than with medicine.

Recently, analysis has awakened from its intellectual slumber. But it still suffers from having showed little or no interest in scientific research until it was too late. Practitioners who had spent years of their lives (and large sums of money) being analyzed themselves had difficulty being critical. Psychiatrists with scientific training gravitated away from the movement. In the last several decades, many of the most effective critics of analytic theory and practice were former analysts who "converted" to the scientific method. Indeed, most contemporary psychoanalysts no longer believe in most of the theories developed by Freud.

When research *has* been conducted on psychoanalysis, it has failed to support cherished ideas (Fisher & Greenberg, 1996). There has, for example, been little support for the concept that childhood experiences shape the development of personality and psychopathology (at least in the way that Freud suggested) (Paris, 2000a). There is little reason to believe that traumatic events are repressed (Pope, 1997). And just about everyone, if asked, can come up with stories describing some kind of childhood trauma. Moreover, most people cope with these experiences and go on to live productive lives. There is no evidence that early adversity is the main cause of any mental disorder, and even in cases where childhood has been abysmal, it does not follow that the best way to deal with the past is to spend years talking to a therapist about it.

Freud's most enduring idea, one that *has* been supported by research, is that there is an unconscious mind. But this does not mean that the unconscious is structured in the way envisioned in psychoanalytic theory. Cognitive theory also postulates mental processes that are not available to consciousness (Stein, 1997; Westen, 1999). This argument does little to support the crumbling edifice of psychoanalytic theory.

Currently, the most influential alternative to Freudian theory is attachment theory. This model, developed by the British analyst John Bowlby (1907–1990), jettisons much of Freud's assumptions and focuses on the long-term effect of the quality (or lack of quality) of the relationship between mother and child (Bowlby, 1969–1980). Attachment theory is also compatible with cognitive models and with developmental psychology. For that reason, it is the one offshoot of psychoanalysis considered respectable in academic circles, and the model has stimulated a large body of good research (Cassidy & Shaver, 1999).

However, attachment theory has pitfalls. First, the way children relate to their mothers does not predict how they will relate to other people as adults. Second, genetic vulnerability can shape abnormal patterns of attachment. Third, attachment theory can be used to support the old mistake (to which psychoanalysis is prone) of blaming parents for mental illness in their children.

Analysts seeking to modernize their discipline sometimes claim that Freud's concepts are consistent with current research in neurobiology (Gabbard, 2000). For example, some recent studies showed that psychotherapy (specifically CBT for obsessive-compulsive disorder) can produce changes in the brain, as measured by imaging (Baxter et al., 1992). When these findings were published, I heard one analyst announce with satisfaction, "We change the brain every day."

One can understand why analysts want to get on the neuroscience bandwagon. But "neuropsychoanalysis" is entirely based on "cherry-picking"—taking the parts of neuroscience that make analysis look good while ignoring the rest. Although one can indeed map emotional responses, both conscious and unconscious, in the brain, this line of research has little to say about theories of psychological development, either those of Freud or those proposed by attachment theorists. Actually, this body of research is much more compatible with cognitive therapy and cognitive neuroscience.

Theoretical problems were not the main reason for the decline of psychoanalysis. A more prominent reason was its failure as a method of therapy: It is time-consuming and very expensive and has never been validated by research. Meanwhile, medicine has changed, and so has psychiatry, with both now requiring that practice be based more on empirical data than on expert opinion. Numerous drugs now have such data showing their effectiveness in treating serious mental illnesses. Psychoanalysis, on the other hand, has no such evidence base, and its failure to develop one has been the source of much disappointment and disillusionment for a generation of psychiatrists who had invested so much time learning and practicing an arduous method of therapy.

Analysts once made great claims for their method of treating severe mental illness (Eisenberg, 1997; Grunbaum, 1984; Hale, 1995). Although Freud was more circumspect about what could be accomplished, his followers often presented the method as a panacea for almost any symptom. Analysts considered their methods to be a sine qua non of therapy—and viewed anything else with contempt. In the 1950s and 1960s, some even claimed that they could cure schizophrenia and other severe mental illnesses, but systematic studies later showed this belief to be entirely unfounded (Dolnick, 1998).

Even today, psychoanalysis has never been properly tested for effectiveness. No data exist, using controlled trials, to tell us whether the length and frequency of psychoanalytic treatment are necessary. The same standards have to be applied as have been used in research on drugs or on other forms of therapy. Indeed, if psychoanalysis were a drug requiring release by the Food and Drug Administration, it would have no chance of approval.

Analysts who are not trained in research methods may quote studies that seem to support their approach. For example, a group of Swedish researchers reported on a large-scale comparison between the long-term outcomes of formal analysis which was superior to long-term analytically oriented therapy (Sandell et al., 2001). However, the absence of an untreated control group made the results impossible to interpret. If you cannot show that analysis is better than brief treatment or no treatment at all, you cannot say anything about its efficacy.

Some have argued that because a proper study of analysis has never been conducted, and because we have no data either for or against the method, we should withhold judgment. But for how long? We are talking about a treatment that has been available for more than a century and yet is *still* unsupported by evidence. It seems unreasonable to wait another hundred years for the evidence to materialize. Moreover, research has supported several cost-effective alternatives to psychoanalysis.

Even in anxiety and mood disorders, the conditions for which psychoanalysis was originally developed, not a single study meeting the standards of scientific research shows analysis to be effective therapy. It is not good enough to rely on "before and after" comparisons. No drug would be allowed on the market on that basis, and no physician would recommend such an arduous and expensive method of treatment on the basis of uncontrolled observations.

There is one final—and ironic—problem with psychoanalysis. Although psychoanalysis, with its broad view of pathology, has the potential to make almost anyone a patient, it was highly selective in practice. Treatment was reserved for patients whose problems were not that severe, many of whom would be considered rather normal. Suitability for this procedure emphasized an ability to function in life; combined with the cost of the treatment, such criteria systematically eliminated patients with disabling mental illnesses.

To counter this objection, a survey was published to show that patients in psychoanalysis meet criteria for DSM diagnoses (Doidge et al., 2002a, 2002b). But, as discussed in Chapter 3, diagnoses prove little, given how many people with normal (or close to normal) functioning can meet criteria for DSM disorders.

The leaders in psychoanalysis (the training analysts) were more likely to treat normal people (many of whom were their colleagues or students), while supervising students on "real" cases. This situation stood in contrast to the medical tradition that the sickest patients should be treated by the physicians with the most experience. Moreover, the length of analysis meant that, unlike other medical specialists, some psychoanalysts might treat no more than 50 people in a lifetime. E. Fuller Torrey, a well-known psychiatric advocate for schizophrenic patients and their families, described this practice as "the abandonment of the mentally ill" (Torrey, 1988).

Today, most young analysts are *not* psychiatrists. Young physicians are not interested in the kind of commitment required for psychoanalytic training when the zeitgeist is against it and their careers will not benefit. (Very few psychoanalysts can make a living from this method alone [Malcolm, 1982].) As psychologists, social workers, and academics from the humanities, many of whom have no training in science, have taken their places, analysts with a medical degree are becoming a rarity, and the influence of psychoanalysis on psychiatry is becoming close to nil.

As a treatment, psychoanalysis can survive only if there is a market for it. The procedure often takes five years, and each year can cost $20,000 and up. Insurance companies do not pay for it. It has to find a niche among people with money who believe that being analyzed is worth this kind of investment. It is still possible to conduct an analytic practice in large cities like New York, but few do this work full-time. Today, given the competition from other briefer and less expensive forms of treatment, psychoanalysis is in real danger of dying out entirely.

Its most likely future lies in modifications of the method for practical use (Gabbard, 2004). For some decades, it has been rare for psychoanalysts to have a patient lie on a couch three to five times a week. Instead, most are treated sitting up, once or twice a week. But like analysis itself, this long-term "psychodynamic" therapy has never been subjected to clinical trials with controls to establish its efficacy. The only serious research has been conducted on brief forms of therapy, lasting a few months—a method different from anything imagined by Freud. By contrast, those of my colleagues who still insist on seeing patients for several years in therapy are not providing an evidence-based treatment. It is possible that some patients benefit from long-term therapy, but we do not know who they are. It is also possible that other patients gain little benefit from extended courses of treatment. It is even possible that some people are damaged by this approach. But without scientific data, we are working in the dark.

Cognitive-Behavioral Therapy

Aaron Beck (1921–), a psychiatrist at the University of Pennsylvania and a recent recipient of the Lasker Prize, U.S. medicine's highest award, was originally trained as a psychoanalyst. He practiced analytic therapy for a few years—until he realized it was not working. He then took his patients off the couch and sat them in an armchair. Beck stopped asking them to free associate and spent less time talking about their childhood and more about their present life. Most importantly, he developed a new set of interventions, which challenged belief systems (negative feelings about future, self, and the world) that make people anxious and depressed. These interventions are what cognitive-behavioral therapy (CBT) is all about. And unlike Freud, Beck conducted rigorous clinical trials from the very beginning to show that his methods worked, results that have been consistently confirmed ever since (Beck, 1986).

Before Beck's research, behavior therapy (BT) was the only competitor for psychoanalysis that was derived from psychological principles. CBT was a conceptual breakthrough that made BT obsolete. Based on the work of the Russian physiologist Ivan Pavlov and the American psychologist B. F. Skinner, BT had proposed that symptoms were learned responses that could easily be unlearned. Hans Eysenck (1973), profiled in Chapter 2, was a strong proponent of BT, which he thought could cure almost any mental disorder in a very short time. However, the data behind that claim were very suspect. Many research studies of BT were based on the treatment of minor problems (such as phobias)—sometimes in volunteers who were not even patients.

What was most troubling about behavior therapy was its total lack of interest in the mind. Behaviorists believed that the mind was nothing but a "black box" and that in the study of behavior one can measure (and consider) only stimulus and response. (These ideas preceded the development of neuroscience methods that have allowed us to look inside the black box.)

Beck, however, brought the mind back by focusing on abnormal thinking patterns. The earlier, BT approach had been unsuitable for the management of depression, a condition in which the main problem lies in mood and thought (not behavior). BT retains more of a niche in the management of anxiety disorders, and therapists still use its methods (e.g., relaxation exercises) for these conditions.

Research data has helped consistently refine CBT, and it has also been applied to problems of more complexity. Although it was originally developed for the treatment of depression and anxiety, CBT is now a "toolbox" that can be applied to almost any disorder. Marsha Linehan, a psychologist at the University of Washington, developed a method of CBT that she calls "dialectical behavior therapy"; it is used for patients with borderline personality disorder who have made repeated suicide attempts (Linehan, 1993). Douglas Turkington, a psychiatrist from Newcastle, UK, has shown that CBT makes a contribution to the treatment of schizophrenia (Turkington, Kingdon, & Weiden, 2006). Recently, techniques for the management of patients with bipolar disorder have undergone successful clinical trials (Scott et al., 2006). Most patients who see psychiatrists can benefit from this (or some other well-structured) form of psychotherapy.

Why CBT Works

The success of CBT has impressed many psychiatrists and other mental health professionals. Hundreds of research studies have demonstrated its efficacy, and it is rapidly filling the niches previously occupied by older therapies. But to be fair, there have been few head-to-head comparisons of CBT and other therapies. In fact, other methods (such as interpersonal therapy, to be discussed below) can be just as effective for conditions like depression (Weissman & Klerman, 1993). Given the large body of evidence (see Chapter 2) supporting the equivalence of most methods of talk therapy, the effects of CBT are probably not unique, but they have been much better documented.

It is instructive to focus on what CBT specifically does *not* do. It does not spend months (or years) sorting out a patient's childhood. That focus contributed to psychoanalysis losing its way. A recent article in the *New York Times* (Spiegel, 2006) highlighting the rise of CBT was entitled "More and More, Favored Psychotherapy Lets Bygones Be Bygones." It argued that cognitive psychotherapists, unlike psychoanalysts, believe that patients should not focus on the past but should put it behind them and address problems in the present. Whenever psychoanalytic therapies or their derivatives have proved at least equal to CBT, they use highly modified methods that incorporate a cognitive approach and focus on the present rather than the past.

In the long run, the greatest contribution of CBT may be that it found a way to maximize the most powerful effects of psychotherapy and to minimize its problems. The most effective elements identified by research as to how therapy works are the "common factors" discussed in Chapter 2. These include high levels of empathy, leading to a good relationship and therapeutic alliance between therapist and patient, and a practical, problem-solving approach to current problems. CBT is designed to maximize all these mechanisms.

I once asked Marsha Linehan, the therapist who pioneered dialectical behavior therapy, whether her method works through common factors. Linehan's reply was, "Yes, but I have found a way to maximize those effects." In other words, CBT focuses on modifying thinking patterns that get people into difficulty, moods that people cannot control, and behaviors that end up being counterproductive.

Like every form of therapy, CBT is a little too much in love with its own technical arsenal. Even if you have a toolbox for everything, that does not prove that tools are the only things that matter. Psychotherapy has always been and will always be a profoundly human experience. CBT may work for reasons other than those suggested by its proponents. We do not actually know that its results depend on correcting distorted cognitions. It is equally possible that it creates a safe haven in which troubled people find new ways to handle problems. What is clear is that CBT makes the good part of therapy work by maximizing common factors.

Currently, CBT is the leading therapeutic "brand name," and even the general public has become aware of the evidence that it is effective. I run an evaluation clinic in a teaching hospital that sees 300 new patients every year. In the last decade, I have rarely seen anyone looking for a psychoanalyst. But many people do ask how they can get CBT.

Although CBT is the most researched form of psychotherapy, it remains the province of clinical psychology, and in spite of intense interest in its ideas, to date relatively few psychiatrists are competent in the method. Its procedures are derived from psychological theories that are not taught in medical school and are somewhat foreign to physicians— psychologists who have been through graduate school are much more comfortable with these ideas. CBT is more like education than it is like medicine: Patients are taught to observe themselves and to change the way they think about their thoughts, their emotions, and their behavior.

Even if psychiatrists were fully trained to conduct CBT, they might not be able to invest the time required to perform it. As noted, psychotherapy can be time-consuming, particularly if patients fail to recover after a few months. Therefore, psychiatrists need to work in teams with psychologists who are trained in the method and have the time to administer it.

On the other hand, CBT's very adaptability—its tools can be used for almost any mental disorder (even if it has not been tested for every category)—has meant that there are now not enough psychologists to provide treatment to patients who can benefit from it. This is unfortunate, particularly now that we have evidence that the method is useful even in the psychoses (not as a primary therapy but as an important adjunct to biological treatment). Its utility here has caused the number of potential patients to rise. Ironically, when psychoanalytic therapy was the main paradigm in psychiatry, there were never enough practitioners to provide it. Now, with CBT, we are similarly hard put to find therapists— unless patients are in a position to pay.

But it is not clear that every psychotherapist needs to be trained in CBT per se, or that this is the only effective form of talk therapy. Short-term psychodynamic psychotherapy (STPP) also has research supporting its efficacy (Dewan, Steenbarger, & Greenberg, 2004). As discussed above, this is a method derived from psychoanalytic principles that focuses more on current problems and usually lasts only 10–20 weeks.

Moreover, interpersonal therapy (IPT) has a scientific base that compares to some extent with that of CBT (Weissman & Klerman, 1993). The late psychiatrist Gerald Klerman (and his epidemiologist wife, Myrna Weissman) originated the method. Although it has psychodynamic roots, IPT might be seen as a manualized form of supportive psychoanalytic therapy, in that it takes a down-to-earth approach to current problems. Klerman, like Beck, started his career as a psychoanalyst but wanted a more practical approach to common symptoms such as anxiety and depression. IPT is very present-oriented but spends less time on modifying belief systems than does CBT, focusing more on practical changes in the patient's current interpersonal relationships.

One gets the impression that there are many other forms of psychotherapy, but only CBT, IPT, and STPP have serious research behind them. Most probably, other methods are variants of these basic types. And even these approaches, which superficially seem to differ, may have a great deal in common.

The Unification of Psychotherapy

One of the great problems with psychotherapy has been the existence of hundreds of types, each defined by its own "brand name," despite often barely noticeable differences in their theoretical underpinnings and practical approaches. But let us imagine a future in which the brand names disappear and there is only one type of therapy, even if it needs to be adapted for different diagnoses. Ideally, such a general form of therapy would maximize common factors and all techniques known to help patients. Thus, psychotherapy would become a unitary discipline with practice based on scientific evidence. That unitary discipline would not require its own name, and every mental health service provider, including psychiatrists, could become well versed in its practice.

A unified field of psychotherapy needs to move beyond an obsession with one method. It is attractive to learn techniques and apply them. But research on psychotherapy has never shown that techniques are crucial. Even for CBT, most of the studies showing that it works compare therapy either to placebo or something called "TAU" (treatment as usual). Thus,

CBT is almost always better than no therapy at all, or the usual mess of clinical management. However, when head-to-head comparisons are made, it is not necessarily better than other methods. I would hesitate to call CBT the "flavor of the month," but trendiness can blind us to the more universal effects of therapy.

Most forms of psychotherapy accomplish the same thing, and the most important elements are common to all methods. Effective therapy is not just a matter of technique but of therapeutic skill. Good therapists get more people better, while mediocre therapists accomplish less.

One thing all evidence-based therapies have in common is that they are brief. When limited to a specific time frame, therapists have to focus on current problems and produce results. Most patients who receive psychotherapy come for a few sessions. "Open-ended" therapies with no time limit can go for years, but that form of treatment is only sought by a very small number of consumers. Effective brief psychotherapy is not that expensive and can be provided to a broad range of patients, but only if professionals are willing to commit themselves to an evidence-based practice and if insurance for a reasonable number of sessions becomes widely available.

In summary, a unitary discipline of talk therapy would integrate all the key components of effectiveness: It would be adaptable to patients' current problems, it would be brief (in most cases), it would be evidence-based, and above all, it would make use of the common factors and techniques that make for a productive therapeutic relationship and would utilize the necessary therapeutic skills required for full effectiveness. To answer the question raised at the beginning of this section, its name would not be CBT, IPT, STPP, or any other legitimate, clinically proven method in the alphabet soup of talk therapy. Its name would simply be *psychotherapy*.

Psychotherapy in Psychiatric Practice

If psychotherapy is effective, why do psychiatrists not practice it more often? One reason is that they are no longer systematically trained to do so. Several years ago, an anthropologist, Tania Luhrmann (2000), wrote a book about the training of psychiatrists, entitled "*Of Two Minds.*" The author described how residency programs no longer teach psychiatrists to conduct extensive courses of psychotherapy, instead concentrating on medicine and pharmacology. Luhrmann was appalled by these changes, but her reaction was to wax nostalgic about psychoanalysis. Her book failed to acknowledge the role of newer talk therapies, such as CBT.

Related to this issue of training, psychiatrists also no longer see psychotherapy as part of their mission—or their fundamental identity. This point of view has infiltrated academic psychiatry, where professors are promoted for research not for clinical skills. Because these same professors make decisions about what gets taught to aspiring young psychiatrists, many future practitioners are not being trained in psychotherapy. Moreover, the mission of psychiatry has changed. Society invests a great deal in the training of physicians, and medical specialists should repay this debt by treating the patients who need the most help— those with severe mental illness. We cannot go back to a time when psychiatrists filled their practices with people suffering from mild problems considered suitable for extensive courses of psychoanalysis. The "good old days" were not so good at all, especially for the patients.

Another factor in the abandonment of psychological treatment by psychiatrists is, in a word, economics. Managed care does not often pay for more than minimal therapy, and health maintenance organizations have become resistant to psychological treatments. In fact, HMOs may insure patients for fewer sessions than we know from research data to be required. (The companies would save money if they paid for more sessions because patients in psychotherapy seek less medical care overall while in treatment [Gabbard, Lazar, Hornberger, & Spiegel, 1997].) Because patients who want to engage in therapy have to pay for it and only a minority of patients can afford to do so, the market drives psychiatrists toward other, more securely funded, tasks. Also, a psychiatrist who sees four to five patients an hour for medication will earn more money than one who spends an entire hour on one patient.

In addition, psychiatrists have been driven out of psychotherapy by competition from other mental health professionals. There is no reason that psychologists and social workers cannot be as competent as (if not more competent than) physicians at providing this treatment. Most therapists now are non-medical, and they generally accept lower fees than physicians do.

Thus, for various reasons, psychiatrists have been moving away from psychotherapy. Although they claim they are still providing psychological services to patients, there is no way of determining the quality of their service. (Chatting for a few minutes before writing a prescription may be a good thing, but it is not psychotherapy.) Fewer psychiatrists maintain active psychotherapy practices, whereas more and more focus on prescribing medication and managing patients in hospitals and clinics (see Chapter 10). This shift has occurred even though psychotherapy is known to be as effective as most other methods.

One might therefore ask whether we should try to turn back the clock and insist that today's psychiatrists be trained to be psychotherapists. As Chapter 10 will argue, psychiatrists, like other highly trained medical specialists, are a scarce resource. They are most needed in emergency rooms, wards, and crisis clinics, providing less direct treatment to patients while spending more time on consultation to psychologists, who are as well trained (and often better trained) in psychotherapy.

All the same, it would be a mistake for psychiatrists to withdraw entirely from the practice of psychotherapy. First, they need experience in these therapies to be able to offer consultations for patients undergoing treatment. If psychiatrists' only unique skill consists of trying out new medications, they will become an endangered species, and perhaps eventually extinct.

Second, even though psychiatrists should focus their treatment efforts on the most complex and severe mental disorders, these conditions also benefit from psychotherapy. While specialized forms of psychological treatment (such as CBT) will largely remain the domain of clinical psychologists, psychiatrists can offer patients brief courses of talk therapy, using evidence-based methods. There is also an advantage when the same person can provide both therapy and medication. Ironically, psychiatrists who understand the limitations of drugs, and who are not worried about "missing something," might be in a better position than some psychologists to prescribe psychotherapy (and avoid prescribing unnecessary medication) for common psychological symptoms.

Third, psychiatric drugs are overused and overrated for common psychological problems. Some patients may recover dramatically with a single prescription—but these are the exceptional cases we like to talk about, not the rule in everyday practice. Many other patients show only a partial response (or no response) to the same medications. Instead of considering psychotherapy as an alternative, today's psychiatrists tend to "adjust" the medication, sometimes on every visit. This is a travesty of scientific medicine.

Finally, psychiatrists with experience doing psychotherapy have a depth of training that helps them be empathic and sensitive with all patients, including those who receive drugs. Even in today's world of brain scans, psychiatrists must not forget how to understand people.

Conclusion

Even if psychoanalytic treatment is not effective for mental illness, we might keep in mind a phrase introduced by Freud's pupil, Theodore Reik (1951), who suggested that therapists help patients more when they "listen with the third ear." Reik was referring to a process of understanding what people feel and knowing what they really mean by what they say. Patients appreciate these listening skills, and science tells us they are an essential element in any type of treatment for mental illness.

Whether or not psychiatrists refer patients for therapy, or provide it themselves, they need to have a sense of how talk therapies should be practiced scientifically. As we have seen, therapists need to be skilled in empathy, patients need to develop a positive relationship with the therapist, and both need to use that relationship to solve current problems. Moreover, most patients looking for therapy should be offered a brief course of treatment that need not last more than six months.

1 0

Psychiatry in Practice

Ultimately, psychiatry must be judged on the services it delivers. No matter how much psychiatrists learn about mental illness and no matter how effective their treatments are, they need to reach the people who need their skills most. In this chapter, I identify problems in the delivery of psychiatric services and suggest ways to improve it.

I have been critical of practice patterns that focus almost exclusively on drug prescriptions. I have also suggested that psychiatrists can integrate evidence-based psychotherapies into their practice, which will provide "added value" for many of the patients they see. Psychologists, social workers, and other health care professionals are already providing the lion's share of psychotherapy services, but psychiatrists should still be familiar with these treatments, have some experience in administering them, and apply them with selected patients.

Each type of mental health professional can be more effective by working in a team. Good mental health care, particularly for patients with severe illnesses, requires collaboration among disciplines. For this reason, office practice is an obsolete way of providing mental health services. Although some psychiatrists are still opening offices for solo practice, an increasing number work in the public health system, with other professionals, where they can coordinate and provide care for the larger community, with its range of mental disorders.

The American system of health care is far from ideal in meeting the mental health needs of its population. Although the United States is the world leader in psychiatric research, it delivers services inconsistently. Most other developed countries, including my adopted country, Canada, have some kind of universal health insurance. (Many offer both public and private care, but most services are insured by a single-payer system.) The United States, in contrast, has a complex system that is a mixture of public care (mainly for the indigent and the elderly), private care (for those who can afford it), and managed care (consisting of privately run insured care with limited benefits). Many people fall through the cracks because they are not well insured or are uninsured. Thus, U.S. physicians (including psychiatrists) practice in a context characterized by fragmentation and unequal access.

Access to services also varies greatly from region to region. A few states have recently required everyone to have health insurance. Yet, in most parts of the country, large numbers of uninsured patients do not have access to high-quality treatment. In fact, many areas lack mental health professionals of any kind. Other regions have many practicing therapists (mostly in coastal cities), located both in clinics and in offices, but even there a psychiatrist is hard to find. In practice, it can be almost impossible to find a psychiatrist who accepts insurance. The United States has more psychiatrists than any other country in the world, but only some people can get to see one.

I will now examine in greater depth what psychiatrists do, where they work, what kind of patients they see, and what their relationships with other mental health professionals are or should be—all in order to better assess, and to suggest improvements in, the various components of the service-delivery system in which psychiatrists play a role.

Patterns of Practice

The American Psychiatric Association (APA) regularly conducts surveys of psychiatric practice in the United States. The National Survey of Psychiatric Practice (NSPP) was conducted in 1998 and repeated in 2002.[1] Both surveys randomly selected psychiatrists from around the

United States. The 1998 survey obtained responses from 71% of those contacted; the 2002 survey had a 53% response rate. (Because the findings of these two surveys are nearly identical, I will discuss them together, with emphasis on more detailed data from 2002.)

The number of physicians practicing psychiatry in the United States has steadily increased over the years. As of 2002 the American Medical Association listed 40,687 psychiatrists. Even though fewer medical students are entering the field, the number of psychiatrists continues to grow. As well, the demographics of psychiatrists are changing. As of 2002, about 73% were men and 27% women, but because the majority of trainees are women, we can expect them to be in the majority of practicing psychiatrists fairly soon. As already noted, psychiatrists are unevenly distributed across the country. Although for every 100,000 persons across the United States, there are 16.5 psychiatrists, New York has 28 per 100,000, Massachusetts 32, and the District of Columbia 57. Some large cities have so many psychiatrists that office practices go unfilled. Meanwhile, rural areas and small towns have almost no access to care.

The surveys show that psychiatrists are spending less time than they used to treating individual patients. On the average, 60% of psychiatrists' time is spent on direct patient care and 20% on administration, with the rest going to consultation, teaching, and research. In comparison to a 1988 survey, direct patient care had decreased (from 67% to 60%), while administration time had increased (from 12% to 20%).

The surveys also showed that psychiatrists are spending less time practicing in private offices. By 2002 only 45% of psychiatrists worked alone, while 28% were located in hospital clinics and 15% were located at inpatient wards. Statistics published in 2006 noted that psychiatric practice had reached a "tipping point" in which public care had become more important than private practice (Ranz et al., 2006).

In the past, psychiatrists worked mainly on a fee-for-service basis. Today their primary source of income is insurance—either from managed care, Medicare, or Medicaid. Psychiatrists who work for hospitals and community clinics may receive salaries that pool such payments. Only 15% of psychiatrists' income is paid directly by patients.

Psychiatrists are not working longer hours but are seeing more patients—on the average, 40 a week. Although the number of patients seen per week has increased, the number of minutes spent with each patient has declined, from 55 to 34. Still the longest time for any medical specialty, half an hour is nevertheless not usually enough time to conduct formal psychotherapy.

Because only 60% of psychiatrists' time is spent on direct care, one can readily see that the classic "50-minute hour" is no longer the dominant pattern. It was noted by the surveyors that psychiatrists make more money (specifically 57% more) by doing three medication checkups than by doing one therapy visit in an hour. That partly explains the decrease in the time psychiatrists are spending on psychotherapy.

Psychiatrists answering the surveys stated they provide psychotherapy to 60% of their patients. That figure does not, however, distinguish between formal sessions based on an established procedure and supportive chats that practitioners might describe as "psychotherapy."

Psychiatrists reported that 76% of their patients are prescribed medication. But this average figure obscures individual differences in practice patterns. Some psychiatrists see most patients in long-term therapy, and prescribe less. Others spend little time talking, but prescribe routinely.

What the surveys do not tell us is who gets to see a psychiatrist. By and large, access depends on economic factors (Wilk, West, Narrow, Rae, & Regier, 2005). Whereas psychiatric consultation and treatment are, at least in theory, available through managed care plans and publicly funded care, specialists are often reluctant to see patients with plans that do not provide adequate coverage.

In summary, these survey results provide a snapshot of a specialty in transition. The office practice of psychiatry is declining, and practitioners are spending more time in public settings. They are treating a larger number of patients and spending less time with each one. The tendency to concentrate on pharmacology has probably had its greatest effect on those entering the field in the last two decades.

Hospital Psychiatry

Psychiatry was born in the mental hospital. A hundred years ago almost all practitioners worked in that setting, which saw a very large number of patients. These jobs were not lucrative, but they were secure. Then, with the development of drugs for severe mental disorders, and with improvements in community services, institutions began to empty (Menninger & Nemiah, 2000).

After World War II, the "separate but equal" status of mental hospitals, which were often located far from other medical centers, began to be seriously questioned. Why should psychiatric patients be treated in a different place and in a different way from medical patients? Was this not an example of stigma? There was talk, soon to become reality, of eliminating most of these hospitals entirely. As patients received effective antipsychotic medication, and as follow-up and psychosocial rehabilitation became available in community mental health centers, many of these hospitals did close their doors. (This was a good thing for most patients, who benefited from living in the community, but some ended up living on the street without any treatment at all.)

At the same time, general hospitals opened their own psychiatric wards and clinics. Because these hospitals treat all kinds of illnesses, many psychiatrists were pleased at a change that reduced the isolation of their specialty. Teaching hospitals attached to medical schools also opened wards and clinics. Before World War II, many medical schools lacked a separate psychiatry department, but by the 1960s all had one (Menninger & Nemiah, 2000).

Still, a gap existed between the mission of the mental hospital and that of a general hospital. When I trained in psychiatry, middle- and upper-class patients (with less severe illnesses) were treated in general hospital wards, while indigent and highly psychotic patients were sent to mental hospitals. Differential treatment of that kind became less common as psychiatric hospitals closed, and today most psychotic patients are admitted to general hospitals. In the United States, when there are not enough paying patients, some remaining psychiatric hospitals actually seek out indigents who are covered by government insurance (Medicaid and Medicare). However, psychiatrists in practice see few patients with that kind of coverage because the government pays much lower fees than private insurers and individuals do.

The large reduction in patients remaining in the hospital means that fewer psychiatrists are required to manage inpatient wards. Admitted patients also have a much shorter stay, partly because treatment is more effective, and partly because managed care plans force psychiatrists to discharge patients earlier.

In fact, as is true for many other medical practitioners, the influence of managed care on treatment has been a major source of irritation for hospital psychiatrists (Regestein, 2000). They feel that their decision making as physicians is held hostage to a bottom line. They are worried that rapid discharge can be bad for patients. On the other hand, psychiatrists are being forced by the system to treat sicker patients, and that is not a bad thing.

A survey led by the distinguished medical sociologist David Mechanic found that patients are actually getting better access to treatment under managed care (Mechanic & Bilder, 2004). Reluctantly, psychiatrists are being forced to change their practice. Although many resent having to discharge patients from the hospital so rapidly, there is no evidence that longer stays are any more effective.

Working in Canada, I do not have to deal with managed care. But government-run medicine has other (and highly effective) ways of controlling physicians' behavior. If doctors keep patients on a ward for too long, cases held over in the emergency room begin to pile up. Given the lack of evidence for longer hospital stays, administrators will badger psychiatrists into quickly sending patients home (which the administrators do, daily).

I am amused when I hear people talk about "checking in" to a hospital. This turn of phrase reflects a past reality, when patients who were not very sick (but had either money or good insurance) could access a bed on an inpatient ward. Today you have to be very sick indeed (either psychotic or seriously suicidal) to get in. Admission to any hospital is a very expensive business. For that reason, it has to be rationed in some way.

Some years ago I was invited by a colleague to lecture at a U.S. university and was given the opportunity to attend morning rounds on one of their wards. The ward was part of a state-run public system that treated patients with little or no insurance, and no one could get in simply because they had money. Nonetheless, my colleague was surprised when I told him that none of the patients we had seen would have been admitted in Canada. Where I practice, the system has developed other ways of managing these acutely ill patients (crisis intervention or day hospitals) that make hospital admission less necessary.

Still, managing inpatient wards remains an essential part of the mission of psychiatry. With the bar raised, most patients who enter the hospital are psychotic and lack insight into their condition. They can be treated only in a controlled setting where medication can be administered and closely monitored. Psychotic patients, in addition to those recovering from serious suicide attempts, are often too sick to remain at home.

Most admissions to hospitals in psychiatry begin in the emergency room (ER). That is where acutely ill people present, and one of the main functions of hospital psychiatrists is to cover the emergency room. This is very hard work. Ideally, the ER would be staffed by a few experienced people, but the job is onerous enough to be unpopular. Thus, duties are often assigned to hospital psychiatrists in rotation. In university hospitals, psychiatric residents (with backup telephone supervision from faculty) usually cover the ER.

Outpatient Psychiatry

Today, psychiatrists spend more time working in outpatient settings. Yet there is surprisingly little published literature describing how these clinics work.

Generally speaking, psychiatrists manage clinic patients who previously might have required long admissions to inpatient wards. As psychiatrists focus more of their energies on the sickest patients, keeping people out of the hospital becomes a major priority. As patients are discharged more often, and earlier, it becomes crucial to maintain patient stability through consistent treatment of outpatients.

At medical schools, outpatient clinics are usually located in a hospital but may also be in community mental health centers. In either case, psychiatrists do not work alone. To keep patients in the community and out of hospitals, we work in collaboration with psychologists, social workers, nurses, and occupational therapists. All these professionals make unique contributions to rehabilitation and therapy, and teamwork produces cumulative results.

Another way to keep acutely ill patients out of the hospital, and one that has been consistently underused, is to offer day treatment. This is an important site of practice rarely described in psychiatric literature. Some of the day hospitals provide "step-down" programs for recently discharged patients; others treat patients instead of having them admitted for inpatient care. Patients come in daily, receive treatment, and go home. This is a practical alternative for patients who are not too sick. Moreover, day hospitals have real advantages in promoting rehabilitation. Psychiatrists are also not under the same tight time constraints that they face on inpatient wards, and one can treat patients in a more leisurely fashion (i.e., in 2–3 months).

The main problem with day treatment is accessibility. Psychiatrists can rarely send a patient directly there from the ER, and admission to wards is much easier. If a psychiatrist is treating an acutely ill patient and wants to make a referral to day treatment, the patient has to go on a waiting list and still has to be followed in a crisis clinic. If patients are not too sick, one can tide them over in this setting, but some patients will still end up being fully admitted.

Outpatient clinics also manage patients for whom hospitalization is not needed, that is, most of the cases psychiatrists see. In general clinics, mood and anxiety disorders predominate, but personality disorders and substance abuse are treated as well. Cases of greater complexity can often be better managed in specialized clinics, where available. These settings have the advantage of applying expertise (and multidisciplinary teams) to treat complex cases meeting criteria for more specific diagnoses. Most medical schools have specialized clinics for schizophrenia, mood disorders, and substance abuse, and they are also useful for personality disorders.

Psychiatrists who work in outpatient clinics face constraints similar to those faced by psychiatrists who run wards and ERs. If you keep patients too long, no one new can get into the system. Human nature being what it is, we get attached to our patients. It is also easier to go on seeing the same patients than it is to evaluate and treat new ones. In the United States, a typical managed care plan allows for monthly visits to a psychiatrist. If a practice is large, there is little pressure to move on to new cases, which would make treatment more accessible. However, because many plans limit the number of psychotherapy sessions, psychiatrists are discouraged from seeing their patients weekly.

In Canada, nobody forces psychiatrists to discharge outpatients, but if too many patients are kept, the system becomes clogged, and the waiting list overflows to the ER (which is where people go if they cannot get an appointment). For this reason, clinic administrators constantly pressure their psychiatrists to discharge patients back to primary care settings and to take on new ones.

The main problem for outpatient psychiatry is the lack of human resources. Even with regular "downloading" of cases to primary care givers and other professionals, there never seem to be enough people to do the work. Psychotherapy becomes thought of as something of a luxury in these settings. In many clinics, brief therapies are available in principle, but access is limited by the availability of professionals trained to administer them. Longer treatments, and specialized methods of psychotherapy, have to be delivered in the private sector.

The absence of long-term treatment (other than medication management) is an important feature of clinics. This fact can create dismay among patients who come looking for psychotherapy. After explaining that therapy is not what we do, I have been asked, "What exactly *do* you do?" I have to explain that psychiatrists treat more severe cases; patients may then ask just how sick they have to be to receive follow-up. The reality—that talk therapy is readily available for those willing to pay—is not what people want to hear. I often see patients who cannot afford (or are not willing to afford) private care but who are looking for treatment in the public sector. But psychotherapy without a fee is rare—both in the United States and in Canada.

In most communities, non-psychiatric therapists are available but are insured only for limited periods. This makes psychotherapy difficult to access. In the absence of this option, patients may see psychiatrists for longer periods of time (albeit less often), if they can—particularly if their symptoms seem to require frequent adjustments of a prescription. What is really happening is that some patients will do what it takes to keep seeing a psychiatrist.

Many of these problems arise because psychiatrists have an unclear mandate. Their skills are increasingly applied exclusively to acute care and the treatment of unstable patients, but many psychiatrists do still follow patients for months to years with a combination of medication management and supportive therapy. In principle, as discussed in the previous chapter, this combination makes for effective treatment for many patients. The problem is that the economics will not support it forever, except in the form of collaborative teams—psychiatrists working increasingly in tandem with other professionals to provide a combination of such treatments to patients on an outpatient basis.

While outpatient clinics often provide good service, access is limited. Patients cannot usually call up and expect to be seen quickly. That is the mandate of the primary care system. And if it takes a month to obtain specialized care, patients who are not being successfully treated either have to wait or have to enter the system by the back door—that is, through the emergency room.

Office Practice

The office practice of psychiatry began in the late 19th century, when neurologists specialized in treating people who had "nervous" problems but did not need hospitalization. Sigmund Freud, who was a neurologist (not a psychiatrist), developed psychoanalysis while running this kind of practice.

Over the course of the ensuing decades, many psychiatrists opened their own offices (Menninger & Nemiah, 2000). This type of practice was particularly congruent with the growing interest in psychotherapy. It was equally consistent with a pattern in which most patients receive a prescription and a chat. In a market with few psychiatrists, it was not difficult to fill a practice. Later, the availability of generous insurance coverage gave office practice great stability. Moreover, office work was always more lucrative than hospital work. Reductions in insurance reversed this situation. The economic viability of office practice devoted to long-term intensive psychotherapy became a problem once managed care arrived.

Practices that mainly consist of psychotherapy can be maintained only as long as there are enough people to pay. Fifty years ago, insurance was not a major factor in psychiatric practice. People were willing to pay out of pocket if they had the money and if they believed they were buying the best treatment. This was a time when patients sought long-term psychotherapy for almost any life problem. (When I was growing up, a local newspaper had an advice column written by a psychiatrist; no matter what the issue, her response always included a recommendation to "go into therapy.") The belief was so strong that when fees went up, patients would be motivated to go into debt or take second jobs to finance their treatment.

In the present climate, one can no longer easily maintain a practice restricted to extended psychotherapy because insurers are not usually willing to pay for it. In Washington, DC, the federal government used to have a generous plan for all its employees, with virtually unlimited coverage that paid for psychotherapies (including formal analysis) lasting for several years (Kiesler, Cummings, & VandenBos, 1979). A few private insurers provided similar benefits. But, eventually, questions about the cost-benefit caused these programs to be cut back or eliminated.

Thus, in the managed care era, office practice has become a more perilous venture for U.S. psychiatrists. They now need to attract referrals of patients who need drug prescriptions; practitioners have gravitated toward this kind of work, which provides a steadier income. By contrast, Canadian practitioners have the option to open an office and to be fully covered under socialized medicine. And yet, my U.S. colleagues have been surprised to hear from me that Canadian psychiatrists do not want to do this kind of work, even when it is fully insured. The loneliness and the difficulties of maintaining a solo practice simply turn most young people away from it.

U.S. psychiatrists who prefer to work alone, especially those who still prefer to provide long-term therapy, can still do so, if they can find patients willing to pay for their services. In urban centers there is a small niche for such paid treatment, and psychiatrists can be divided into those who take insurance and those who do not. But in most places, only a few have enough wealthy patients to practice that way.

In summary, although solo office work still accounts for almost half of total activity among psychiatrists, that figure is likely to decline in the coming years. Again, economic factors are strangling that kind of practice, with managed care putting a cap on the number of times patients can be seen. Above and beyond the issue of economics, however, is office practice even the right model for 21st-century psychiatry? A practice that focuses mainly on office visits and prescriptions does not always provide the best service. When practitioners work alone, patients have no access to the skills that psychiatrists lack. Much more can be accomplished in a team. Moreover, office practice was developed for healthier populations and is not the most efficient way to deliver services to sicker patients.

How Many Psychiatrists Does Society Need?

Psychiatrists are expensive. It takes a long time to train one—four years of medical school, followed by four to five years of specialty training. The fact that psychiatrists are physicians means that their training will cost more than that of other mental health professionals. It also means they are a scarce resource.

Given this circumstance, what is the unique role that only psychiatrists can fill? Family doctors (and internists in general practice) can and do prescribe medication for certain mental health conditions. In fact, more patients today receive antidepressants from family doctors than from specialists (Sareen, Cox, Afifi, Yu, & Stein, 2005). As for psycho-therapy, psychiatrists have lots of competition. Clinical psychologists provide much more psychotherapy than psychiatrists do, and many social workers have active therapy practices. Although there is wide variability in training (and exposure to evidence-based treatments), there is no evidence that psychiatrists are better therapists.

The one arena where psychiatrists remain indispensable is the hospital, where the sickest cases are. Psychiatrists are still needed to run inpatient wards, to staff emergency rooms, and to treat the most fragile patients in outpatient clinics. But given these apparently limited confines requiring unique psychiatric expertise, does the United States, which has the world's highest ratio of psychiatrists to the general population, need so many specialists, particularly if most of them work only in some areas of the country?

The supply of psychiatrists reflects the large number of medical schools and residency programs in the United States, and the fact that the country continually imports practitioners from abroad. Are all these highly and expensively trained specialists really needed, now or in the future?

It is in a balanced assessment of supply and demand that we must define the role and mission of psychiatrists today and tomorrow. In the service of that redefined role and mission, we must mandate that psychiatrists be better educated and better trained in *all aspects* of the current understanding, diagnosis, and treatment of all mental disorders. We must also require that more enter practice and provide services as concentrated, targeted specialists working solely in tandem with other mental health and medical providers, especially in acute care.

The 41,000-plus specialists we have now will never be enough if they have to provide all services by themselves. But these numbers might well be sufficient if psychiatrists work in teams with other professionals.

To meet their debt to society, specialists have to be available to meet the burden of mental illness. That burden is real even after one takes into account the overestimates that DSM-driven epidemiological studies of various mental illnesses have generated in recent years.

But the 41,000-plus psychiatrists are not all we have. Once we factor in contributions of psychologists and social workers, the picture looks quite different. Meeting the mental health needs of the population does not depend on medical specialists alone. It would be a great mistake for psychiatry to "defend its turf" against competitors. Patients benefit when professionals from many disciplines are involved in and work together for their care. Psychiatrists may have specific expertise in psychopharmacology, but they can accomplish more and extend their effect on mental health by performing more consultations.

The precise number of psychiatrists needed by society, as estimated by health planners worldwide, has varied greatly between countries or even within countries (Faulkner & Goldman, 1997; Feil, Welch, & Fisher, 1993; Weissman, 1996). The reason is that these estimates depend on the role that psychiatrists are expected to take.

In a market system, such as the U.S. model, the number of psychiatrists could continue to increase until it reaches saturation. But, such a concentration would not address the real problem: What kinds of human resources, and which skills, are needed to manage mental illness in the population?

Shared Care

In hospitals, every medical and surgical ward has consultation-liaison psychiatrists to advise physicians. Similar consultations for patients being seen by other professionals are available in outpatient clinics. These activities offer a model for a different vision of psychiatric practice.

Perhaps the most important type of consultation that psychiatrists can and increasingly will provide is to family doctors. As with internists, family doctors usually see patients before specialists do, often providing biological treatments for mood and anxiety disorders without necessarily understanding what they are prescribing. Their patients benefit more when these "first-line" practitioners regularly work with psychiatrists.

These consultations are the basis of a system called "shared care" (Kates et al., 2006). This term refers to a mode of practice in which family doctors treat most patients—but with strong and consistent support and backup from specialists. With proper training and consultation, there is no reason that family physicians cannot manage common mental disorders more often.

In a shared care system, psychiatrists are involved in the treatment of many more patients than in a system in which they work alone. (The model can also be extended to nurse practitioners, who are now allowed to prescribe in many jurisdictions, and to professionals, such as psychologists and social workers, who usually cannot prescribe but who treat many sick people.)

As more patients that psychiatrists treated in the past are successfully managed instead by family doctors, the main focus of psychiatric practice will be on the treatment-resistant cases and on the most seriously ill.

Even so, family doctors with extra training and support can also look after many, if not most, of the chronic patients psychiatrists have always seen (i.e., those with schizophrenia and severe mood disorders receiving long-term medication). Chronic patients need specialist care when acutely ill, but when they stabilize, their medications can be maintained by non-specialists. Although family doctors are sometimes reluctant to treat the severely mentally ill, they can be made comfortable by readily available specialist backup.

Thus, for shared care to be effective, it has to offer rapid (ideally same-day) consultation for family doctors when trouble arises and things go wrong. The knowledge that expert support is available when needed allows non-specialists to carry even very difficult cases. Some psychiatrists have experimented with spending time in multidisciplinary primary care clinics, where they can talk directly to their physician consultees (Kates et al., 2006). The most important need, they found, is for a rapid response, whether by telephone or in person. (Another possibility is "telemedicine," with video consultation.)

The value of a well-managed consultation cannot be overstated. The very process of obtaining an expert opinion is vastly reassuring for consultees, even if there is nothing further to be done for the patient. And in many cases, consultation leads to changes in both diagnosis and treatment that improve a patient's status. When expert opinion is readily available, family doctors can develop a competence that approaches that of the specialist in many domains.

One of the most common scenarios I see concerns patients who have been prescribed multiple antidepressants but show no improvement. As a consulting psychiatrist, I try to help family physicians get off the medication treadmill. (Few are aware of the STAR*D study.) I also bring psychosocial stressors to their attention and suggest ways in which patients can receive community support in addition to (or instead of) a purely pharmaceutical regime. (The main reason doctors cannot effectively make these recommendations to their patients is that there is a lack of psychotherapists whose fees people can afford.)

I can describe several other common scenarios that require expert consultations. One concerns patients who express suicidal ideas. There may be some cases in which the presence of a serious mental disorder such as melancholic depression would require specialist care. But most of the time, the psychiatrist's task involves reassuring the family doctor that suicidal thoughts are common symptoms (which by themselves should not be considered cause for alarm). Another common complaint, particularly these days, is mood swings. The task of the psychiatrist is to determine whether a bipolar disorder is present or (more commonly) whether mood instability has another cause. The scenario that might arouse the greatest concern is one in which patients appear to be either developing a psychosis or else relapsing in the presence of a chronic psychotic disorder. Although a simple adjustment of medication might sometimes be sufficient, these are the cases that often need to be treated by a specialist, at least until the patient is stable.

The United States needs to find a way to better train family doctors in the delivery of good basic mental health services. One could imagine a future in which, increasingly, primary care attends to most of a patient's needs, but the patient has access to specialists on referral. That is the way the system works in other countries—as well as those parts of the United States where few specialists practice (Kates et al., 2006). Direct access to a specialist is only common in urban settings.

The main obstacle to such a change is the reluctance of medical school graduates to choose family practice as a profession. It is more difficult to carry out practice in which one has to more or less know everything than it is to pursue a specialty. Moreover, most specialties pay better.

Another problem is that family doctors, like all physicians, are dependent on a fee-for-service system. The more patients you see, the more you make, even if the system is hardly conducive to the care that most patients require.

It is easy to write a prescription for an antidepressant. But who is going to take the time to make sure the patient takes it regularly? (Many patients stop during the first week because of side effects.) And who is going to provide the psychotherapy that depressed patients need? We do not know the quality of care patients receive when prescribed an antidepressant by a family physician or an internist. Psychiatrists could therefore usefully spend more time than they do now consulting with these professionals and providing courses for them. Also, family doctors, like psychiatrists, are limited in what they can deliver when they work alone. They, too, might accomplish more by working in multidisciplinary teams.

Working in Teams

Psychiatrists cannot deliver comprehensive service unless they work cooperatively in a team with psychologists, nurses, occupational therapists, and social workers, each of them knowledgeable enough to know when to call in the services the others can expertly provide—be they medical management or psychotherapy or psychosocial rehab or a combination. These teams can also include primary care physicians.

The role of psychiatrists in these teams would not be limited, as it often is now, to the writing of drug prescriptions. They would provide regular and easily available consultation on diagnosis and treatment. They would also be involved in direct care of the most difficult patients, whether that involves drugs or psychotherapy. Medical specialists, who are uniquely qualified to assess psychopathology and to guide the provision of treatments of all kinds, would play a leadership role.

Teams following this model already exist in hospital clinics, particularly those that focus on the treatment of the sickest patients, such as those with schizophrenia. Most patients attending these clinics are assigned to another mental health professional; meanwhile, the psychiatrist looks after the prescription, while always remaining available for consultation in a crisis or when treatment review is indicated. But psychiatrists in these teams also provide direct care for the most unstable cases.

In many ways, the evolution of psychiatry from solo practice to a team approach has already begun. Many psychiatrists already do perform a crucial consulting for other physicians and for other mental health professionals. This trend needs to be extended so that teamwork becomes their primary mode of operation, and direct care focuses on acute and severely ill patients. Thus, they would apply their expertise to the sickest patients (who need to see a specialist) and to the wider range of patients who see other therapists but can benefit from expertise in diagnosis and triage to select the best treatment.

This vision stands in contrast to the way specialists in psychiatry work now, especially when they practice alone in an office. On the whole, solo psychiatric practice has become a prescription only for prescriptions—and little else.

Psychiatrists, Psychologists, and Social Workers

The distinctions in training between psychiatrists and clinical psychologists produce differences in the ways they approach practice. Trained first as physicians and then, after obtaining their medical degree, as specialists in mental illness, psychiatrists increasingly focus on medical forms of treatment. By contrast, psychologists obtain a master's or a doctorate, which enables them to become either academics who teach or do research, or practitioners who, after internship training, can treat patients. Those who become practitioners (i.e., clinical psychologists) generally specialize in psychotherapy. For example, cognitive-behavioral models of therapy, although first developed by a psychiatrist, have had greater impact in clinical psychology, which has been committed to evidence-based practice longer than psychiatry has.

That said, some psychologists believe they should be allowed to prescribe medication. In 2002 this practice was allowed (with certain restrictions) in New Mexico (Yager, 2002). The main argument for doing this was that the state had a shortage of psychiatrists, and patients would receive better care if psychologists could write prescriptions. It might also be argued that psychologists are more likely to spend time with patients than are family doctors. Follow-up research on the effects of this social experiment would be valuable but has not yet been carried out.

This policy could increase access to medical care but might make it even more difficult for patients to get psychotherapy, especially if psychologists, like psychiatrists, find they can make more money by seeing more patients in a short time by prescribing medication. Ideology and economics would drive practice. Even now, some psychologists have arrangements with physicians to put most of their patients on drugs. If they were allowed to prescribe, the practice of psychologists might end up resembling that of psychiatrists.

Thus, letting psychologists prescribe could mean that even *more* people who do not really need medication will be given it, and a bad situation could get even worse. Patients will probably benefit more if psychologists concentrate on what they are trained for without trying to assume the role of psychiatrists. In communities where psychiatrists are unavailable, patients can receive medication from family physicians.

Social workers have developed their own model of psychotherapy, which they have traditionally called "case work." Unfortunately, this kind of therapy, even if helpful, is not evidence-based insofar as clinical trials have never been part of the social work tradition (Weissman, 1996). Nonetheless, case work provides support, comfort, and practical help for many clients.

Social workers also have a different spin on mental illness. Traditionally, they have been less interested in diagnosis and more interested in functioning. Psychiatrists might have something to learn about a point of view that promotes health and personal strengths rather than one that focuses on eliminating illness.

Psychiatrists already work closely with social workers in hospital settings and outpatient clinics. These professionals are essential for managing patients with chronic illnesses, such as psychoses, where rehabilitation is the focus. Market forces have also encouraged social workers to carry out psychological treatment. In family therapy, although many of the pioneers in the field were psychiatrists, social workers came to dominate. In individual psychotherapy, social workers have opened their own practices. Still, when social workers require a consultation, they need access to psychiatrists.

Again, the best model for treatment is multidisciplinary teams, where psychiatrists, psychologists, and other professionals work together. The main obstacle is the limited number of professionals in all categories. It takes money to provide good, professional care. Unfortunately, mental health is usually at the bottom of the list of priorities for governments and insurance companies. The situation is even worse in small towns and rural areas, where mental health clinics may not even exist.

The Future of Psychiatric Practice

In summary, for psychiatrists to play a role in the larger mental health mission, they may have to give up practicing in offices and work in hospitals and clinics. This is already the trend in the field, driven in large part by the managed care system, but other factors contribute as well. The current mental health care system suffers from serious problems with access to care. There will never be enough psychiatrists to manage the needs of all mental health patients (from the mildest to the most severe cases). This is why psychiatrists need to work increasingly as consultants to other physicians and to other mental health professionals, in shared care models. This may be the only way for psychiatrists to deliver their unique skills to the large number of people requiring mental health services.

For this model to become truly effective, the current system for delivery of services in the United States will need to change. Described in a 2003 presidential commission report as "fragmented," the U.S. mental health care system is resistant to change because economic interests (those of psychiatrists in managed care companies) still dominate.[2] Another reason for resistance is cultural—the traditional U.S. resistance to bureaucracy and regulation.

Nonetheless, to meet the needs of the large population, health care may have to be even more regulated than it is today. U.S. society does not believe in central planning, and it has left the distribution of services to be determined by market forces. Although the market remains the best way to create wealth, it is not necessarily the best way to provide services. If health is considered a basic right of all citizens, then governments need to do some planning. (We would not, for example, accept a totally unregulated school system.)

I am not suggesting that universal health care with a single payer would be a panacea. I have had too much experience in Canada with bureaucrats whose ignorance about grassroots needs is infuriating. (Moreover, the waiting list problem is real.) Canada has a socialized system, but governments give little priority to mental illness. When they do intervene, their priorities are political, not medical. In the Canadian system, government ministries spend money on dialysis, artificial hearts, and high-tech cancer treatments, while routinely starving less expensive mental health services. Canada had its own federal commission on mental health, but when it came time to decide on how to provide money for more services, the best it could come up with was a proposal for an extra tax on alcohol (Kondro, 2002). (Needless to say, that idea went nowhere.)

Nonetheless, options from across the border might still be better than the current U.S. system, which costs more and accomplishes less for the greatest number of people than do systems in other developed countries.

The U.S. presidential commission report made some recommendations for improving the situation in mental health, but they were vague. For example, it put great emphasis on reducing the stigma of mental illness. There is no doubt that doing this would remove one of the most important obstacles to improving services. But accomplishing that goal is not simple. Except for organizations like the National Alliance on Mental Illness (NAMI), there are few advocates for patients with mental illnesses and their families, who have little influence on public policy. Lack of influence means less money and fewer services.

The APA has been actively lobbying for "parity" in insurance coverage, that is, the end of discriminatory practices that make it more difficult to get mental health care than other types of treatment. The best argument for such a change is that accessibility to care for mental disorders actually *saves* money—by reducing the demand for unnecessary medical testing and treatment (Gabbard, 2004).

How can we ever hope to develop a more rational system in which psychiatrists can practice? I do not think the changes I have suggested here will happen by fiat, but they could emerge through a process of evolution. As health care becomes more expensive, costs have to be contained. Better access could be one of the "side effects" of that process.

Conclusion

As demand for mental health services goes up, there are more unsatisfied customers who are asking for better care. Patients and their families often complain about insensitive psychiatrists who over-prescribe medications and about the unavailability of psychotherapy. At some point, there will be enough public pressure to force the mental health system to be properly funded and to provide treatment more rationally.

In the meantime, psychiatrists need to keep their eyes on their mission. Unfortunately, the economic health care system in the United States works against public health. Psychiatrists suffer economically if they treat sicker patients who are not well insured, if they carry out more consultations, and if they do fewer medication checkups. Although I do not foresee immediate or dramatic changes in the U.S. system, it will probably evolve into a model in which minimal access for everyone is guaranteed. If that happens, psychiatrists would be in a better position to provide evidence-based care for the patients who need it most.

PART IV

OUTLOOK

1 1

Training Psychiatrists

I completed my residency training in 1972. As I prepared to go into practice, the divisions within my specialty, discussed throughout this book, troubled me. I had some teachers who believed that talk therapies offered the best treatment for mental illness and others who believed that drugs were more effective and should replace psychotherapies. Because most teachers had radically different points of view regarding the best approach to treatment, students like me had to make our own choices.

I wanted to be an all-around psychiatrist with a wide range of skills; I was deeply interested in psychotherapy (although I rejected the narrow vision of psychoanalysis). I also learned to prescribe drugs to treat patients with severe mental disorders. But my main ambition was to be a teacher. I wanted to bridge the gap between the two camps of psychiatry and teach a new generation how to be comfortable and competent in both worlds. This goal has proved harder to achieve than I ever anticipated.

With time, I came to realize that psychiatry did not know enough about mental illness to provide effective treatment consistently. That is why I eventually became a researcher. I benefited from a broad education, and psychiatry gave me the chance to pursue rich and varied careers as physician, psychotherapist, teacher, researcher, author, editor, and administrator. I remain happy with my decision to enter psychiatry, and I still encourage young people to make it their life's work. The obstacles toward achieving that goal are many, however, beginning, of course, with those one encounters in medical school.

Medical School

Every psychiatrist has to train as a physician, but in the four years of medical school little time is given to the study of mental illness. Medical students attend only a few lectures on psychiatry and spend between four and eight weeks in wards and clinics. The culture of medical school is dominated by internal medicine and surgery. For example, students spend much more time learning how to manage heart disease and cancer than they do learning about treating mental illness. Although these priorities are understandable, they make the transition to psychiatry difficult.

Choosing psychiatry as a specialty requires medical students to go against the grain. The decision to enter the field is often questioned by teachers and peers. That remains true today. Medical students may get a negative reaction from their teachers when they inform them they have chosen psychiatry. They also may hear demoralizing comments suggesting that psychiatrists are not real doctors.

This negative image of psychiatry within medicine is in part the consequence of its past failures. For many years, the discipline was slow to adopt the scientific standards that have shaped modern medicine. Because it is now doing much better in this regard, it is better accepted and respected by those in other medical disciplines.

But there is another, perhaps deeper, problem plaguing psychiatry. Mental illness itself carries a stigma, and many physicians have the same negative attitudes to the mentally ill as does society in general. Even though mental disorders are among the most common conditions found in medicine, physicians often see them as a kind of moral failure and as problems patients should be able to control themselves. In these circles, depressed people can be described as lazy and therapy is dismissed as merely "hand-holding."

In the 1960s psychiatry was a much more popular choice for medical students than it is today. The very factors that lowered its estimation in the eyes of medicine (its humanistic approach to suffering) made it attractive to many young doctors like me. At that time, a medical student with a humanist bent had almost *no choice* but to be a psychiatrist. (Family practice was not yet a common option.) As noted in Chapter 2, fewer medical students are choosing to specialize in psychiatry (Sierles et al., 2003; Sierles & Taylor, 1995). Ironically, the field became less popular as it became more scientific.

What further complicates recruitment is the fact that psychiatry is not always taught well in medical school. Rotations that last only a few weeks in medical school rarely provide students with the experience of looking after patients. Moreover, medical schools may not expose students to the most interesting and relevant aspects of the field. Many programs place students on inpatient wards, settings where all patients have severe illnesses. A student's role in this setting is mostly as an observer, and many students get the false and off-putting impression that psychiatrists look after untreatable cases most of the time.

It would make more sense to train medical students on patients they are likely to see later in their careers—whether they go into psychiatry or not. Patients with common and less severe problems come to outpatient clinics. When medical students are taught psychiatry in these settings, they find the experience more interesting. However, outpatient placements require close supervision and much more faculty time—time that most faculty do not have.

Another problem is that the psychiatrists who educate medical students are rarely academics. Not all faculty members are interested in teaching medical students. The most ambitious researchers are usually too busy to teach, and when they do teach, they would rather spend time with residents committed to their specialty. Clinical teachers may be highly enthusiastic but are not always up to date on evidence-based medicine.

Students who apply to medical school with the idea of going into psychiatry (I was one of these) are more likely to explore the field despite the shortcomings of medical school. But some students will never have thought of psychiatry until they are exposed to it in medical school. They may find themselves surprisingly fascinated with mental illness and are more likely to commit to psychiatry if they are exposed to charismatic teachers and if they have the chance to learn about new and exciting developments in the field.

Not all residents come to psychiatry directly from medical school. Some come to psychiatry from other medical practices, particularly family medicine. Family physicians treat many patients with psychological problems, and some feel it is only natural for them to become specialists.

A fair number of international medical graduates (IMGs) go into psychiatry as well. The American Psychiatric Association (APA) surveys discussed in Chapter 10 show that IMGs now comprise 40% of psychiatrists in the United States. Although these graduates can be as bright and as skilled as any native-born physician, few medical schools in the developing world meet North American standards. In some countries, students may never have had experience treating patients before graduating. Physicians who have trained in such settings sometimes have a lot to learn, even if they pass a standard examination allowing them to do residency training in North America: Not all physicians from abroad, for example, have a thorough understanding of the uniquely cultural dimensions of their North American patients' experience.

In view of all the problems associated with the weak exposure to psychiatry in medical school and the fact that psychiatrists do not make as much money as other medical specialists do, it seems we should be *happy* that as many as 2–3% of students choose psychiatry and that there are still enough interested students to fill most residency programs. Clearly, the quest to understand diseases of the mind retains appeal, but interest might be even greater if medical schools invested a bit more in fostering it.

Psychiatric Training

The transition from medical school to postgraduate training in psychiatry requires a period of adjustment. Once residency training begins, many students discover that most of what they learned in four years of medical school is, with some exceptions, no longer relevant. Trainees have to accept that a residency in psychiatry feels like starting from scratch.

In fact, there has been much discussion among educators about how much general medicine should be included in a psychiatric residency. In the 1970s many programs had no requirement for an internship. But psychiatry wanted to ensure that it was seen as a medical specialty like any other. For this (largely political) reason, the rules were changed, and many programs either required their residents to do a full year of training in other specialties, or mixed psychiatry with other specialties in the first year of training (Varan, Noiseux, Fleisher, Tomita, & Leverette, 2001).

Over the years, I have heard many opinions about the relative effectiveness of internships versus no internships, but I have seen little solid evidence to support one model over another. In fact, nobody has ever compared the ultimate competence of psychiatrists trained in one system to that of those trained in another to find evidence of the superiority of a particular educational approach; they instead rely on educators' opinions.

My own view is that training residents in the traditional internship, outside psychiatry, adds little to the skills of practitioners. In Canada, there was for many years no requirement for further medical training within the psychiatric residency. Many colleagues trained under that system are now middle-aged. These psychiatrists know as much about medicine as anyone else. Working as consultants to medical and surgical wards forces them to keep current. Wherever they work, they use as much internal medicine and neurology as they need. Whatever they end up doing, they have to learn most of it on the job.

It can be argued that taking care of sick people as interns will instill medical knowledge in psychiatrists. But because medical students today take a much more active role in patient care than they did in the past, those entering residency have already gained that firsthand knowledge. Also, psychiatric residents get plenty of experience looking after medical problems in their own patients. For example, if they prescribe drugs (like atypical neuroleptics) that produce metabolic problems, they will have to relearn some endocrinology. In the Canadian system, we assign residents to spend four to six months within their first year in family practice clinics (Varan et al., 2001). This makes more sense than spending time on medical wards because family doctors are typically the ones seeking psychiatric consultations, and they see the most common psychiatric conditions.

I would guess that no more than 10% of the education psychiatrists receive in medical school is of any practical use. With the exception of practitioners who specialize in consultations for other physicians, most psychiatrists treat a select population and quickly learn the complications of the drugs they use. In outpatient clinics, where I have worked for most of my life, psychiatrists see a wide variety of patients and need a solid knowledge of medicine to understand the effects of medications that patients have received from other physicians. But again, they learn most of this on the job.

What medical training provides psychiatrists is the ability to pick up non-psychiatric but undiagnosed illnesses. When this happens, we all feel good about ourselves. But in all the years I have practiced, I have seen only a few cases like that. Of course, my experience reflects the kind of work I do (community consultation), and medical comorbidity is much more important for a psychiatrist working in a geriatric clinic or in con-sultation-liaison.

In summary, we do not know what kind of training produces the best psychiatrists. But even though the required medical education is es-sential for those practicing psychiatry, much of what we learn will never be used. We will never again be asked to treat pneumonia or kidney failure. For this reason, spending additional time on medical and surgical wards during an internship seems less likely to be helpful than exposure to primary care would be.

Finally, there are many tasks that psychiatrists are expected to per-form for which they receive no training at all. How do you learn to be an inspiring teacher, a helpful consultant, or a competent administrator? The answer is that one mostly learns on the job; no amount of training, especially in areas outside one's specialty, can prepare one for every aspect of the task. Of course, it helps to have some natural talent, and mentorship is always important.

Residency Training

How do we prepare future psychiatrists for the complex roles they will be expected to assume? One thing we have to do is ensure that trainees are exposed to a wide variety of clinical settings. All programs require that psychiatrists in residency training spend some time on inpatient wards, and in outpatient clinics, and that they do regular night call in the emergency room. In most hospitals, this structure guarantees that resi-dents will be exposed to a wide variety of patients. In each of these settings, residents will be closely supervised, usually on a one-to-one basis.

The exact mix of requirements for clinical training varies, and there is an important difference between Canada and the United States. In Canada (as in Britain), all programs are run directly by universities (not hospitals). Programs arc accredited by a national organization that monitors them closely and designs all details of the program. There are additional specific requirements (every resident must spend time in child psychiatry, geriatric psychiatry, consultation-liaison psychiatry, and re-habilitation). Moreover, residents are required to train at more than one hospital. In Canada, residency lasts five years, not four. (For those with a fellowship in a subspecialty, the total is six years.)

In the United States, traditions of local autonomy have always been strong. Thus, psychiatric hospitals are free to set up their own residency programs (which may be only loosely affiliated with a medical school). While there are accreditation procedures, they are not always followed closely. A typical four-year training concentrates on general psychiatry. If students want to do specialized work, they need to apply for a fellowship. Also, child psychiatry in the United States is a separate specialty, like pediatrics, with its own fellowship program and its own exams.

The U.S. system is, like so much else in the United States, good for the best, and bad for the worst. Not all hospitals teach a full range of skills or have a representative mix of patients. The most prestigious residency programs are located at top-level universities. At these top centers for training and research, one need not worry about getting a second-best education. However, not every program meets the same standards. Psychiatric hospitals, for example, may not be the ideal site for complete training. The quality of residency training differs among institutions, and when the entire training is in one hospital, residents tend to get a skewed view of psychiatry. Also, not all residents at psychiatric hospitals are exposed to researchers and serious academics, which has consequences for their ability to conduct evidence-based practice. It would be better if such programs offered joint training with general hospitals.

Because the model of training in residency is one of apprenticeship, the quality of a residency program depends on the commitment of its educators. On a human level, aspiring psychiatrists are often attracted to the teachers who spend the most time with them and take a personal interest in them. But this does not ensure good training. In addition to being accessible, teachers must also be aware of the latest developments and pass their knowledge on to students. Unfortunately, not all faculty members who love teaching are committed to a scientific, evidence-based psychiatry. The paradox of residency, as with so many other educational settings, is that researchers have less time for teaching, leaving students to spend more time with clinical faculty who may or may not be up to date on the latest research.

There is no guarantee that this dilemma will be solved any time soon, so students must learn to fend for themselves. Thus, psychiatric residents need to learn to read the literature on their own. One established method for training students to understand scientific articles is "journal club." This is a regular meeting at which residents review a recent scientific paper and participate in a critical discussion about it. I have been running journal clubs for 35 years and have seen how they help trainees become comfortable with published data. Once students become familiar with statistics, tables, and all the data of serious science, high-level journals are no longer daunting. Critical reading is now being taught in medical schools to enable residents to arrive with some mastery of journal reading.

Another question about psychiatric training is how much time should be spent teaching biological treatments and how much should be spent on talk therapies. Since psychopharmacology now primarily defines what psychiatrists do, education today puts great weight on how to prescribe drugs. By contrast, psychiatrists are receiving inadequate training in psychotherapy. In the past, psychoanalysts dominated top residency programs, and competency in long-term psychotherapy was considered a sine qua non for training. The triumph of biological psychiatry marginalized these skills.

But analytically oriented psychiatrists still retain some clout in residency education. The Residency Review Committee (an accrediting body for U.S. programs) recently recommended that all training should produce psychiatrists who are at least "competent" in psychodynamic (i.e., psychoanalytical) psychotherapy (Mellman, 2006). This misguided ruling does not seem to consider whether that form of psychotherapy has a strong evidence base. It also fails to consider that other methods do. It would have made more sense to demand competence in psychotherapy without specifying that it be based on psychoanalysis.

It is also not clear what this requirement will mean in reality, and it may be more honored in the breach than in the observance. If you do not have the right teachers, you cannot offer supervision for effective psychotherapy. In my own department, I tried to encourage the residency program to teach evidence-based methods such as cognitive and interpersonal therapy, not just analytically oriented treatment. However, since we still had many more psychoanalysts than faculty trained in other methods, the possibilities were limited.

As the office practice of psychotherapy by psychiatrists is declining, and as practitioners spend more time on medication management, competence in talk therapies may not be an outcome that educators still consider essential. (Even so, a recent survey found that psychiatrists receive more formal training in evidence-based psychotherapies, such as cognitive and interpersonal therapy, than do clinical psychologists and social workers [Weissman et al., 2006].)

Once training is complete, examinations are held, supervised by a national organization, the American Board of Psychiatry and Neurology. The exam consists of a multiple-choice section plus an oral exam (part of which requires a brief interview with a patient). Most residents pass the boards. But unlike in Canada and Britain, psychiatrists in the United States can practice without passing an exam. Certification nonetheless provides prestige and is usually necessary for an academic position.

Preparing for Practice

Residency in psychiatry is based in hospitals and clinics, and psychiatrists who plan to continue to work in these settings should be well prepared for their careers. But those who choose to work alone in an office practice have to learn another set of skills. This is why the annual meeting of the APA offers training sessions on how to open an office. Even if solo office practice is becoming anachronistic within psychiatry, it remains an option for graduates. Physicians have a long history of independence and entrepreneurship, with privileges closely guarded by the American Medical Association. Many practitioners love their autonomy and prefer not to work in a university or a hospital.

Moreover, the number of psychiatrists who complete residency every year is large, and not all can find good jobs in hospitals and clinics. In Canada, the numbers of graduates are rigidly controlled (although under socialized medicine, everyone earns a good income immediately after residency). Office practice in Canada has almost disappeared (except in two or three large cities), and almost all young psychiatrists work in institutional settings.

Another decision that young psychiatrists have to make is where to work. Like other professionals, most prefer to live in urban areas. This is one reason that people outside large cities lack access to psychiatrists. In Canada, residents are required to spend part of their residency in rural areas (Hodges, Rubin, Cooke, Parker, & Adlaf, 2006). These regulations are intended to encourage psychiatrists to work there, but the requirement does not seem to have the intended effect. Some provinces have actually tried to force young people (by not insuring them) to live outside cities.

Psychiatrists affiliated with universities are needed to educate medical students and residents. But in teaching hospitals linked to universities, clinical psychiatrists, although part of the academic mission, are not provided with an office to practice. Another pattern (found at a few U.S. universities but more common in Canada) is for all psychiatrists to be either full-time or close to full-time, in which case they do *all* their work in a hospital office. Either way, most faculty teach part-time. And even today quite a few psychiatrists who teach residents are committed psychotherapists.

Full-time faculty are more likely to be researchers with a biological bent. They may not see many patients. Only a few psychiatrists become tenured academics—and there will never be more than a few. Even if one earns a salary from the university, the money is much less than one can earn in practice.

Although academics would like to recruit more residents to research careers, it is understandable that few choose this route (and that many drop out along the way). Researchers live in a highly competitive environment in which one lives and dies by grants and publications. You have to have a thick skin to deal with rejection (which is the fate of most grants, and most submitted papers). Compared with research, treating patients provides almost instant gratification.

Continuing Medical Education

Once psychiatrists go into practice, they may or may not keep up with current literature. Not everyone has strong intellectual curiosity, and not everyone has the time (or the inclination) to read journals. Moreover, clinical practice does not reinforce a scientific worldview. Given this circumstance, coupled with the rapid changes that have occurred in medical practice, physicians in most jurisdictions are now required to prove that they are participating in continuing medical education

(CME), which allows psychiatrists to collect credit points for a variety of activities. They earn most of their points by attending conferences where CME workshops are offered, like the annual APA meeting, or by attending local events to which prominent speakers are invited.

Many CME activities are funded by the pharmaceutical industry. A certain percentage of the money the companies provide for this purpose is "unrestricted," in the sense that hospitals and universities have the right to choose their own speakers. But the industry often prefers to bring in its own speakers, who directly or indirectly promote their latest products.

CME for psychiatrists is designed to encourage lifelong education in a changing field. Yet, although learning styles differ, most adults do not find that listening to lectures is the best way to learn. Physicians who attend conferences remember very little of what they hear there. By comparison, pharmaceutical representatives visiting psychiatrists in their places of work provide information (or misinformation) on a personal basis in manageable doses, thereby potentially having a greater effect on practice.

Although CME is a good idea, there has been no systematic effort to monitor its effectiveness. We need research to determine whether physicians actually change their practice as a result of attending conferences. And CME may have even less effect on those who need it most—solo practitioners. Psychiatrists may be less motivated to keep up with developments in their field when they work alone. Even if you earn your credits, you may not integrate this knowledge into practice. One learns more by working with stimulating colleagues, which is why institutionally based specialists are more likely to be current.

Conclusion

Young psychiatrists will determine the future of the field, so what they are taught is critical—from their days in medical school to their days as practitioners. What theoretical information should they be exposed to? Should they be learning more about neuroscience? What kind of clinical experience should every future psychiatrist have? Should psychiatrists be competent in psychotherapy?

The proper emphasis in psychiatric training will continue to be debated, but what makes psychiatry fascinating is that the best practitioners need to know a bit of everything—from neurons to the human condition. Psychiatrists need skills in biological treatment, in psychotherapy, and in managing the social context of illness. Yet teachers of residents do not always take such a broad view. Psychiatrists, even in top universities, are being trained only in a narrow biological model that enables them to be competent in the prescription of drugs.

That said, new models of psychiatric practice will likely open doors that the decline of psychotherapy and rise of neuroscience have closed. As young psychiatrists become expert consultants, they will have a greater, and a more rounded, impact on mental health services.

Psychiatry and Society

A t one time, the media would ask psychiatrists to prognosticate about every problem under the sun. After all, they were supposed to be experts on the *mind*. In one famous incident, for example, a group of psychiatrists opposed the candidacy of Barry Goldwater for president in 1964 because they believed that his political views provided evidence of his mental instability. Even now, psychiatric opinion in the public arena is routinely solicited, especially after a terrible event. Osama bin Laden was described as mentally disordered in the weeks following 9/11, and every witness of that horrific day was primed in the media to be at risk for posttraumatic stress disorder (PTSD). More recently, in the days following the events at Virginia Tech during which a student gunned down more than 30 students and faculty before killing himself, the media interviewed several psychiatrists about what may have contributed to a murderous state of mind. Diagnoses ranging from paranoid schizophrenia to antisocial personality disorder to PTSD issued forth from psychiatrists on the evening news, none of whom knew the young man as a patient. (If they had known him, patient confidentiality would have dictated silence.)

Psychiatric diagnosis requires gathering very specific information about patients, and psychiatrists' attempts to diagnose people they have never met are arrogant and foolish. (They would also be unwise to put friends or family members in DSM categories—however much they might be tempted to do so.) Psychiatrists learn about patients in a clinical setting and should be satisfied to be medical specialists who treat sick patients. I hope that will always be the case.

But the temptation remains for psychiatrists to give their opinions on all kinds of issues, publicly and privately, even when these opinions are not scientifically based. For example, some psychiatrists think they know the best methods for raising children. In fact, when it comes to childcare, everyone has an opinion, and pretensions to omniscience about the upbringing of children are not limited to clinicians. A researcher I know has studied maternal care in rodents and, based on that experience, has pontificated for the media about how mothers should treat babies. As this case suggests, it is all too tempting to go beyond scientific evidence to prescribe the "right" behaviors for everyone.

Even within their professional lives, psychiatrists are routinely asked to go outside their expertise. Employers and insurance companies ask them, for example, to fill out medical forms excusing people from work. I am reluctant to do this because I know that patients with similar symptoms remain at their jobs. The same principle applies to university students seeking to be excused for missed exams and late papers. (I worked in a student mental health service for 25 years and almost always refused to provide such excuses. The letters I did write simply stated that students had attended the clinic, but sympathetic professors used them as valid excuses anyway.)

Physicians can certainly see themselves as advocates outside the clinical realm, but doing so can carry a social cost. In this chapter, I examine the ways in which psychiatrists are asked to offer their expertise to various societal institutions. I argue that the role of the psychiatrist is solely that of a physician dedicated to the treatment of mental illness and that psychiatrists should not expand, or be asked to expand, this role to include legal or social matters outside their realm of knowledge. I also suggest that, in the public health domain, psychiatrists should not concentrate on the prevention of mental illness until research has been undertaken to show that prevention is actually possible.

Psychiatrists as Expert Witnesses

Providing expert testimony in the courts is the most visible aspect of the social role of psychiatry.[1] Society asks for medical opinions from psychiatrists about a number of legal issues. When should people charged with criminal offenses be excused on the grounds of mental illness? Should people suffering from physical injuries receive compensation for psychological injuries? What arrangements for care are in the best interests of children? If providing a medical opinion were the only thing psychiatrists did in the courtroom, expert testimony would be unproblematic. But psychiatrists sometimes take positions in court that say more about their personal values than about scientific expertise.

I have never testified in court myself (and hope I never have to). But I once took a course from an expert in the field on how to behave on the witness stand. What troubled me about the instructor was that he accepted that psychiatrists are asked to resolve issues beyond their medical competence. I asked him why we should agree to answer them. His reply was, "If we don't, who will?"

Views on philosophical issues such as the mind-body problem and reductionism influence how psychiatrists treat patients. In the courtroom, another philosophical question arises—do we believe in free will and moral choice, or in psychic determinism? Everyone agrees that people who are flagrantly psychotic have lost some degree of free will and cannot make moral choices in the same way. But the questions that psychiatrists are asked by the legal system are often in a gray zone.

Bias derived from personal values becomes a problem in a field like psychiatry, where scientific knowledge remains thin. What seems to be medical opinion may reflect only the expert's perspective on the human condition. Lawyers can usually find psychiatrists to take either side on the question of criminal responsibility. This leads to conflicting testimony in a "battle of experts." Courts (and juries) may be inclined to discount expert testimony entirely.

Experts are not necessarily objective and, like any human being, are subject to biases. Some forensic psychiatrists almost always testify for the prosecution in a criminal trial, whereas others almost always testify for the defense. For example, in high-profile cases, from that of John Hinckley (who shot President Reagan) to that of Andrea Yates (who killed her five children), the same forensic psychiatrist testified on the side of the prosecution. Does this witness believe that people are, with rare exceptions, responsible for their actions?

On the other hand, many psychiatrists tend to underplay free will and moral choice in favor of some form of psychic determinism. That bias might incline us more to support the defense in criminal cases. As a profession, we see behavior as determined, whether by genes or by upbringing or, increasingly these days, by a combination of both. It follows that forces outside the control of the individual must drive criminal acts. In the past, expert witnesses sometimes tried to present defendants as victims of an unhappy childhood. These days, a better strategy is to claim that people accused of crimes have a mental disorder and acted as they did because of a chemical imbalance.

Consider this example. Chapter 4 discussed the infrequently used DSM diagnosis "intermittent explosive disorder." Defense lawyers have attempted to frame impulsive violence as a consequence of this condition, and expert witnesses have told courts not to hold a defendant responsible—if his serotonin levels made him do it. This "serotonin" defense has actually been advertised on the Internet by a law firm.[2]

The argument is based on a statistical relationship but downplays the absence of evidence for any *predictable* link between brain serotonin levels and violence. Most people with low levels are never violent, and among violent populations, there are only a few cases in which serotonin is actually low (Krakowski, 2003). Fortunately, this type of defense has yet to catch on.

Another currently popular defense in criminal cases is the diagnosis of bipolar disorder. As we have seen, this condition can be diagnosed on very slim grounds. A few years ago in Canada, a high profile politician's career ended when he was caught stealing an expensive ring (intended as a present for his lover). However, criminal charges were dropped when the politician's therapist testified that he was suffering from bipolar disorder (even though the defendant, who was in psychotherapy, was receiving no medication for such a condition).

The vast expansion of psychiatric diagnosis allows almost all aberrations of behavior to be considered a feature of mental illness. This trend has created grounds for determinism that can be exploited in the courtroom. If DSM diagnoses were routinely considered defenses for criminal behavior, the entire legal system would collapse.

The Insanity Defense

Psychiatrists have been providing expert testimony in criminal trials for more than a century and a half. In such cases, they may be asked to give an opinion on an insanity defense.[3] This practice started in 1843 with the case of Daniel McNaughton, who murdered the secretary of the British prime minister (confusing this man with his employer, who McNaughton thought was persecuting him). McNaughton's delusional ideas led the court to declare him "not guilty by reason of insanity." Even today, the basic principle behind any insanity defense is usually some variant of the "McNaughton rule," that is, that a defendant could not distinguish right from wrong at the time he committed the crime.

The insanity defense has always been controversial. In a 1954 case, a liberal judge (David Bazelon) proposed a broader rule, suggesting that "an accused is not criminally responsible if his unlawful act was the product of mental disease." This "Durham rule" took its name from the burglar, Monte Durham (a 23-year-old man who had been in and out of jails and mental hospitals for most of his life), whose appeal produced the rule.

The Durham rule was applied only in one jurisdiction (Washington, DC) but may have increased the number of people committed to St. Elizabeths Hospital in the following years because people who might otherwise have gone to prison were sent to a psychiatric ward. Yet no one can determine whether criminal actions are a "product" of disease, insofar as most people with mental illnesses never commit crimes. We may agree that alcoholism and drug addiction are disorders, but we do not accept these diagnoses as the basis of an insanity defense. Moreover, surveys of prisoners show they have a high rate of mental disorders (Hodgins, 2001).

Since then, other rules have been proposed as the basis for an insanity defense. In 1972 the American Law Institute recommended it be based on a defendant's lacking "substantial capacity either to appreciate the criminality of his conduct or to conform his conduct to the requirements of the law." The vagueness of this standard is fairly obvious, and the proposal never caught on. In 1984 Congress passed an act that suggested an insanity defense must present "clear and convincing evidence that at the time of the commission of the acts constituting the offense, the defendant, as a result of a severe mental disease or defect, was unable to appreciate the nature and quality or the wrongfulness of his acts." (If anyone knows what "clear and convincing" means, please tell me!) The rest of the wording of this proposal goes right back to the McNaughton rule.

One of the major problems with the insanity defense is that expert witnesses are unable to support their opinions with brain scans and blood tests, so they have to rely on observation and opinion. That seemed to change during the most famous insanity defense in U.S. history. The trial for John Hinckley, who attempted to assassinate President Ronald Reagan in 1981, was held in Washington, DC, and the outcome, which outraged many, may have been determined by a quirk in the law in that district that put the onus on the prosecution to *disprove* insanity—rather than requiring the defense to prove it.[4] As a result, Hinckley remains in a hospital rather than in a prison.

The Hinckley defense was the first to introduce a brain scan to support an insanity defense. Hinckley's lawyers had expert psychiatrists who argued that he suffered from schizophrenia, and the defendant's CAT scans were entered as exhibits. The scans showed a certain degree of shrinkage of the cerebral hemispheres, a change that can be seen in schizophrenia. However, shrinkage is not specific to the disease and can occur in perfectly normal people—a discrepancy that experts for the prosecution noted.

The defense may have succeeded in the Hinckley trial, but the fact remains that there is no biological test for schizophrenia. Even if there were, the question of moral responsibility would still stand. Although mentally ill people are statistically more likely to commit violent acts, most people with schizophrenia never hurt anyone. Therefore, we cannot assume that the disease is the cause and that crime is the effect. Again, determinism is tempting but simplistic.

Psychiatric Testimony and Civil Law

Although few psychiatrists are called to testify in a criminal trial (that job is reserved for experts, with most witnesses being forensic specialists who do this kind of work full-time), many psychiatrists do testify in civil cases during the course of their careers. Yet requests for psychiatric testimony in civil law are not necessarily based on medical knowledge. Many requests concern the custody of children, in which psychiatrists are not particularly expert. Moreover, questions about custody only rarely depend on diagnoses of mental illness.

The closest I ever came to being dragged into court is when I was subpoenaed in a custody dispute in which a mother had been evaluated in my clinic. I had found no mental disorder, so I got out of the situation by informing the lawyer that if he forced me to testify, I might be a hostile witness. The only time I would have happily testified involved a man with bipolar disorder who had been brought under control with lithium but who was still barred by his wife from seeing his children.

In these disputes, the courts would be better advised to obtain testimony from social workers. In a case where psychiatric testimony was requested by a court before returning an abused child to its mother, I asked the worker on the case why her observations, based on her visits to the home, were not more relevant than those of the psychiatrist. She said that judges believe more in the expertise of physicians than of social workers.

Personal injury cases are another common setting for expert testimony. Psychiatrists may be asked to estimate the amount of psychological damage an individual sustained in an accident. Although one could argue that this kind of work is necessary, it is not apparent to me why psychiatrists (and not accountants) should be asked to do it. Nothing in our training prepares us for putting a dollar sign on disability. And there is nothing evidence-based about such a procedure.

Psychiatrists are not always neutral experts in the courtroom, and they are not necessarily expected to tell the truth. Because they are paid for their testimony, and their employers are lawyers who represent one side in an adversarial system, they usually end up saying what these lawyers want them to say. This is why psychiatric expert witnesses are sometimes referred to as "hired guns" and why I believe they should refuse to take part under such circumstances.

Expert testimony pays very well, so it is easy to see how economics can drive psychiatrists away from their mission to treat patients. I am sad to say that I know colleagues who see fewer patients because they can earn much more money as expert witnesses. Most people act to maximize their income, but physicians have a different responsibility. More than anything, these choices involve a moral judgment.

Social Psychiatry

Most of this book has focused on the struggle between biological and psychological models of psychiatry, but there is a third way to look at mental disorders and their treatment. This third model, social psychiatry, links mental illness to social influences and emphasizes prevention rather than cure. It addresses questions not considered in biological or psychological models, instead proposing that social factors are implicated in the causes of mental illness and can influence their course and outcome and affect service utilization (Eisenberg, 2004). (The related field of transcultural psychiatry examines how ethnicity and culture affects mental illness—in our own society, and in other parts of the world [Murphy, 1982].) Social psychiatry is unique in that its links are less with medicine than with the social sciences: particularly with sociology, which studies how social support (or the lack of it) can affect mental health, and with anthropology, which describes cultures in which the prevalence of mental disorders is different from our own.[5]

Social psychiatry was most influential in the 1960s, when the theory that mental illness was caused by cultural and social forces was at its height. Psychiatrists dedicated to this model suggested that we should take society—not just individuals—on as a "patient." This view has been overshadowed in recent years by developments in neuroscience. In an article published in 2004, however, Leon Eisenberg proposed a synthesis. Addressing the perception that genetics and biology have made social psychiatry obsolete, he noted that genes do not determine behavior. The influence of biology is to "bend the twig," not to determine the precise shape of the tree. The final shape of the illness is influenced by social forces.

We have three ways of showing that social factors affect mental illness (Paris, 1996). First, some disorders are more common in specific socioeconomic classes (usually lower ones). Low socioeconomic status has a strong influence on disease, poverty being bad for health. But it is also possible that people vulnerable to mental disorders are more likely to end up poor. Research on schizophrenia demonstrates how difficult it is to sort out this problem. As a biological illness, it often leads to poverty and unemployment. But schizophrenia is also more common among disadvantaged ethnic groups, independent of income, in immigrant populations. It is unusually common among West Indian immigrants in the United Kingdom, for example, and among Moroccan immigrants in Holland (Cantor-Graae, 2007). This suggests that the social stressors associated with living in a foreign culture may, for some who are vulnerable, have a role in the expression of the disease.

Second, disorders can be more common in some cultures than in others. Unless there are genetic differences between groups, these findings show that culture can have a direct effect on risk for mental illness. A good example is substance abuse, which varies greatly from one society to another (Helzer & Canino, 1992). Some mental disorders are fully "culture-bound," that is, they are seen *only* in some societies and not in others (e.g., eating disorders are unheard of in cultures where there is not enough to eat [Szmukler, Dare, & Treasure, 1995]).

Third, some disorders have become more prevalent over time. For example, rates of depression, substance abuse, and suicide have all increased among young people since World War II (Rutter & Smith, 1995). Because gene frequencies do not change in just a few decades, but social circumstances do, this kind of data provides strong evidence for social influence.

The explanation is that social structures promote certain kinds of mental disorders and suppress others (Paris, 1996). In modern societies, there are stressful social demands that can trigger symptoms in vulnerable individuals. Although all societies have mental disorders, people who have support from extended families and traditional communities may be protected to some extent because social roles are defined by the community. For example, in societies where marriages are arranged, no one need live outside a family. In some societies, people have the same jobs as their parents; their societal roles are laid out for them and they do not have to find an "identity" or worry about unemployment. These issues can eliminate certain stress factors that promote certain kinds of mental illnesses. On the other hand, they may add different sets of stress factors that promote other mental illnesses.

In the same way, individuals in the same society and facing the same stress factors but having different personality types may be affected differently. In other words, social networks and intimacy depend on context. For example, shy people tend to do better in a stable traditional culture where they hardly ever meet someone they do not know. Therefore, social phobia can be thought of in similar terms as asthma—a problem that is rare under some conditions but has become more common due to environmental changes (Wakefield, Horwitz, & Schmitz, 2005).

Any rapid change in prevalence occurring over relatively brief periods of time is likely to reflect social causation, at least in part. Mood disorders, and rates of attempted and completed suicide, vary widely from one culture to another and have greatly increased in North American society since World War II (Rutter & Smith, 1995). How mood disorders are defined does, of course, influence these prevalence rates, but suicide figures are more factual. Eating disorders develop under specific cultural conditions (i.e., when food is abundant but young people are expected to be slim) (Szmukler, Dare, & Treasure, 1995). Borderline personality disorder, associated with overdoses and self-cutting, emerges with modernization and social change (Paris, 1996; Walsh & Klein, 2003).

The importance of social context does not in any way contradict the biological and psychological realities of mental illness. But even the course of the most serious disorders differs from one society to another (Paris, 1996). For example, although psychoses are universal, patients are less likely to recover from them in large cities, where they are more likely to become isolated and jobless, than in rural areas, where many can still find social roles (Murphy, 1982). But social influences probably have their greatest effect on those who are vulnerable for other reasons.

Psychiatrists, of course, have to practice in their own culture and cannot control prevalent social risk factors. Our main purpose as psychiatrists is to treat mental illness, however it is caused or exacerbated, and to relieve our patients' suffering.

Can Psychiatrists Prevent Mental Illness?

The last example of psychiatrists' social role concerns the question of whether we can apply data from social psychiatry (and other domains) to the large public health issues surrounding the prevention of mental illness. It might even be possible to use genetic data in the future to identify those at risk for disease and to prevent mental disorders. Prevention has often had dramatic effects; vaccination against infectious diseases is one example. But one needs to know something about what causes a disease before one can prevent it.

The idea of preventing mental illness had its heyday during the hegemony of psychoanalysis. At that time many psychiatrists thought they understood the causes of mental disorders, believing many conditions to be the result of bad parenting. It followed that we could prevent illness by teaching mothers how to raise their children. Widespread belief that good mothering produces mentally healthy children explains why Benjamin Spock's book on childcare was so popular.

That idea was a vast illusion. People can become mentally ill despite excellent parenting. Moreover, since resilience to adversity is ubiquitous, many people can grow up perfectly normal in spite of exposure to terrible parenting. Further, it has been proved that, among those who are biologically vulnerable, the relationship between childhood trauma and adult mental disorder arises from gene–environment interactions (Paris, 2000a). In that respect, a biological perspective on mental illness has relieved families of unnecessary and unmerited guilt.

In the past, resistance to biological psychiatry came from psychotherapists who thought that if something was genetic, a patient's fate was almost entirely predetermined. Today we know this is not true—genes express themselves only under specific environmental circumstances. DNA is not destiny. Even if you have a parent with a psychotic illness, you are unlikely to develop the same condition (McGorry & Singh, 1995).

Child psychiatrists, understandably, are interested in the idea of prevention, and some of them entered this subspecialty with the hope of preventing adult disorders by treating children early. But again, evidence for effective prevention is lacking. Only a few findings (mainly involving educating parents about setting rules and limits) suggest that interventions can decrease the prevalence of behavioral disorders in children (Brestan & Eyberg, 1998). Although common sense suggests that parents can be taught to prevent conduct disorder in a child, we have very little solid data to support this idea. Existing findings, drawn from small-scale research, do not justify expending money on large-scale programs to teach parents.

The idea of prevention in psychiatry has traditionally been associated with political liberalism—the belief that by fixing social and political structures we can prevent or cure mental illness. Thus, in the 1960s goals of social change underlay the community psychiatry movement. In its minimalist version, community psychiatry set reachable goals—keeping patients out of hospitals and making sure that everyone had access to treatment for mental problems. But in its maximalist version, community psychiatry claimed to have special knowledge and expertise to guide the creation of better families and a better society to prevent mental disorders.

This idea proved illusory—or rather, it was upended by disillusion with social engineering. Psychiatrists do not know enough about the causes of mental disorders to prevent them. And the concepts behind the community psychiatry movement were particularly naïve in failing to take into account the biological basis of mental illness. Like psychoanalysts, community psychiatrists championed their ideas even though they lacked evidence to support their claims. The ethos of the 1960s was one of high hopes—even if the belief in prevention eventually led to disillusionment and reaction.

Although everyone agrees with the principle that to prevent is better than to cure, interventions to prevent mental illness must be supported by data. We should no more accept the idea that a particular approach can prevent illness without subjecting it to proof (through clinical trials) than accept an unproven form of treatment.

There is actually very little evidence that serious mental disorders can be prevented. There is only some evidence that milder problems, such as depressive symptoms or childhood behavioral problems, can be ameliorated by simple interventions early in life (Kazdin, 2006; Schoevers et al., 2006). But there is no reason to believe that psychiatrists know how to prevent psychoses, substance abuse, or serious mood and anxiety disorders.

I doubt that many psychiatrists today spend much time thinking about the prevention of mental illness. That should not be seen as neglect. Until prevention becomes evidence-based through systematic research, we would be wrong to invest in interventions that are unproven, however well meaning.

Moreover, even when we know that social stressors cause mental disorders, there may be little that psychiatrists can do. Suicide is a good example (Paris, 2006b). There can be little doubt that social forces influence the frequency of suicide. Rates vary between genders, among occupations and social classes, and from one country to another. And suicide is a major public health problem (the 11th most common cause of death at all ages, and the 2nd most common in young adults). Yet, as discussed in Chapter 7, no one has ever demonstrated that methods of suicide prevention can be widely effective. Many interventions have been tried—the most widespread include educating physicians and other key "gatekeepers" to refer patients for treatment, and closely monitoring patients who have made suicide attempts. The problem is that most people who attempt suicide succeed the first time. Suicides are usually men who die by shooting or hanging. No one knows how to prevent these people from killing themselves. Psychiatrists cannot eliminate social stressors in a person's life; their expertise lies in identifying and treating illness once it develops.

Conclusion

Psychiatry has a larger social dimension than other medical specialties do, but the temptation to recruit psychiatrists to solve all of society's woes, whether in the legal system or in other areas, is unfortunate. Because psychiatrists do not know what causes mental disease, their theories outside of medicine reflect prejudices rather than concrete knowledge. These prejudices also reflect widely held societal beliefs. Some beliefs may be well meaning; others, such as the belief that we know the "right way" to raise children, are misguided. Psychiatry cannot compromise its mission of helping sick people by basing its opinions on unscientific beliefs. Only a large body of new knowledge could make it possible for psychiatrists to undertake the evidence-based prevention of mental illness.

The Future of Psychiatry

A Story of Extremes

Psychiatry has gone from one extreme to another throughout its history. At one time it was famous for promoting fantastic psychological theories that had no basis in science. Many psychiatrists were spending their careers conducting office practices, providing psychotherapy to patients who were unhappy but not ill—the so-called worried well. These practitioners did little hospital work, rarely prescribed drugs, and used little medical knowledge.

Psychiatrists were unhappy with this situation. They craved the respect, prestige, and certitude of other fields of medicine. At the same time, many psychiatrists were disillusioned with psychoanalysis, which had failed to keep its promises as a radical cure for mental illness and which had little support in research. With the development of effective drugs for mental illness, psychiatry believed it had the opportunity to solidify itself as a medical science.

Beginning in the 1970s, psychiatry fell in love with neuroscience. Now the field is dominated by biological theories, and psychiatrists mainly use drugs to treat patients. The romance and excitement of our field today lies not in dreams and free associations but rather in genes and brain scans. Psychiatrists long for the day when their field will have as accurate a picture of the illnesses they treat as other physicians have of their fields' diseases. Unfortunately, this wish has had the undesirable consequence that patients (and even people who are not sick) are being overmedicated. In contemporary practice, patients and psychiatrists seem to be convinced that medication is the answer to every problem. Because of this, an entire method of treatment (psychotherapy) is considered outmoded, and training in psychotherapy has decreased significantly.

Psychiatry has gone to extremes and needs to regain its balance. The current state of the field is a great improvement over the past, when diagnosis was mostly a matter of opinion, and effective drugs had not yet been developed. But to make further progress, we need to adopt a broader model, one that does not reduce the mind to molecules. We also need to look at the past and place our current problems in the context of history.

The Historical Context of Modern Psychiatry

Medicine in the early part of the 20th century was almost as mysterious as psychiatry is today. The basic functions of the organs of the body were understood, and pathologists had carefully studied how their appearance (and microscopic structure) changed throughout the course of disease. However, the precise mechanisms by which disease developed were still obscure. The main exceptions were bacterial infections, whose role in disease had been established in the previous century. The most serious problem was that therapeutics remained in a primitive state and physicians rarely cured patients.

It is interesting to examine the *Textbook of Medicine,* the field's standard text, written by the leading medical academician of the time, Sir William Osler (1898), and published in several editions at the beginning of the 20th century. No contemporary reader can help but be struck by the fact that the less that was known about a disease's pathology, the more theories were proposed to explain it. But at least Osler was committed to finding scientific explanations for these puzzling conditions. Although experimental medicine and clinical trials lay decades in the future, Osler always remained open to new ideas and eschewed dogmatism.

A hundred years ago, psychiatry faced even greater problems. Psychiatrists who adhered to a medical model did not have enough data to support it. Sigmund Freud became prominent because he proposed to fill a vast vacuum of knowledge. The famous German psychiatrist Emil Kraepelin, considered the leader of his discipline in Europe for his books on psychoses, had to depend entirely on clinical observation rather than the measurement of disease processes. He was like a man in a darkened room trying to figure out where he was by bumping into the furniture.

Osler is still revered for his methods, but his book is antiquated. As psychiatry advances, today's textbooks will be equally out of date. I often wonder what psychiatrists in 50 or 100 years will think of today's psychiatric textbooks. In fact our specialty is just beginning its journey. By the end of the current century, the diagnosis and treatment of mental illness will have changed as much as it did in the past century.

Unfortunately, psychiatrists and their patients are in no position to wait for future miracles. The current lack of knowledge about the causes of mental illness tempts psychiatrists to cling to theories that are unproven. Although today it is unlikely that a charismatic doctor could promulgate a dubious treatment through enthusiasm alone, physicians are still susceptible to faddish ideas. When a treatment is dramatically effective with some patients, it tends to be tried on many others. Thus, the problems associated with psychiatric diagnosis are not issues for academic hair-splitting. They have real consequences for how patients are treated.

Psychiatry keeps changing its mind. As a student, I entered a specialty dominated by psychoanalysis. In the 1960s I observed the rise (and fall) of the community psychiatry movement, which Roy Grinker (1964) once described as "psychiatry galloping off madly in all directions." Then, as early as the 1970s, I knew psychiatrists who believed that every human problem could be cured by medication. Along the way, I have lived through a vast array of therapeutic trends affecting assessment and treatment.

Fads and Facts in Psychiatry

Perhaps because psychiatry is my field, I notice its susceptibility to fads more than that of other medical specialties. Nonetheless, it does suffer from a less well-developed understanding of the causes of illness than do other fields of medicine. And because of this lack of knowledge, it is more susceptible to shifting and often unfounded theories and treatments—that is, to trendy ways of thinking about, diagnosing, and treating mental illness.

But fads are usually based, at least in part, on facts; it is the way that these facts, sometimes very meager in number, are used that produces these trends. Hence, because facts about the causes of mental illnesses are so thin, we attempt to fill our gaps in knowledge with conjecture about what might work to treat a given patient with a given mental illness: If it happens to work in Patient A, then maybe it will work in Patients B through Z.

Still, psychiatry is not the only medical field susceptible to such tendencies. Medicine as a whole has never been immune to fads. Fads are tempting because physicians have always been, and still are, unable to treat many diseases. And so they and their patients have resorted to questionable therapies for conditions that have no established means of treatment. Thus, alternative medicine flourishes for untreatable diseases (witness the continued appeal of dubious therapies for terminal cancer). On the other hand, hardly anyone would ask an alternative medicine practitioner to remove an appendix or manage a bout of pneumonia. Yet, concerning matters of mood and behavior, people are more willing to accept unproven treatments.

Fads also result because psychiatrists spend most of their time treating patients with chronic diseases, where quick and easy success is rare. Today patients usually see psychiatrists because they have shown resistance to treatment by family doctors, who have taken over the management of mild depression and panic disorder, and by psychologists, nurses, and social workers, who administer most forms of psychotherapy. Psychiatrists and patients alike want to end the patient's suffering, and it can be tempting to hope that any treatment which shows promise of success will be a silver bullet.

Physicians also pride themselves on being up to date. Even when there is a standard accepted method of therapy, they may be tempted by "the latest thing." (This is why the pharmaceutical industry does so well in marketing new drugs.) Yet doctors are often better off sticking to older forms of treatment until newer ones are proved by evidence-based research to be effective. After all, medicine has had many false starts and false hopes, and past experience shows that many trendy treatments proved useless.

By and large, medicine as a profession attracts people who want to *do* something, actively. Academics and researchers are trained to question everything and demand proof. But physicians are more like soldiers, preferring action to doubt. (I would like to think that psychiatrists are a little more thoughtful than most physicians, but our track record does not justify this conclusion.) Moreover, medical schools do not always train doctors to think critically. Although medical curricula have been reformed over the years so that most graduates have learned how to read the scientific literature, the problem of failing to think critically has not been eliminated.

Neuroscience and the Future

Despite my rejection of the idea that psychiatry is nothing more than applied neuroscience, I agree that practice will eventually benefit from brain research. In the long run, as neuroscience unlocks the secrets of the brain, patients with mental disorders will receive more effective treatment. In this respect, I agree with writers who look forward to a biological future for the field (Hobson & Leonard, 2001). I have emphasized in this book that psychiatry suffers from the absence of biological markers to identify disease processes. This is the reason that psychiatric diagnoses, which are based on observational data rather than on underlying processes, continue to lack validity. Psychiatric treatments, which target symptoms rather than disease mechanisms, are largely "shotgun" approaches. If we could measure what is going on in the brain, we could use that information to monitor treatment.

But no matter how advanced the technology of the future, patients will still need to be treated by professionals who care about their minds and about *them* as human beings. And there is nothing more complex in science than the study of the mind. For this reason, we cannot practice in expectation of future breakthroughs but rather must base our practice on what we do and do not know *now* about the brain, and what we do and do not know *now* about the human mind and the human condition. The struggle for the future of psychiatry should ultimately turn on what helps patients most. Psychoanalysis fell from favor because it failed as a therapy. Drugs stepped into the breach because they worked—at least for some groups of patients. Our current over-reliance on medication reflects a lack of practical alternatives. In the future we will probably do better.

In the meantime, we should not fall for the promotions of the pharmaceutical industry. Psychiatrists do not have dramatically better treatment methods than they had 25 years ago. Nor should the public expect breakthroughs in drug therapy in the near future. Even if brain research is on the march, advances in treatment do not move lockstep with advances in science. Some of the greatest discoveries in psycho-pharmacology occurred by accident, and we still do not know how most psychiatric drugs work.

In summary, even the greatest discoveries in neuroscience have not led to better treatment in the short run. The long-term outlook is more hopeful. Better and genetically targeted drugs with more specific actions are likely to be developed. Also, electroconvulsive therapy, an effective treatment that works by stimulating a large number of brain neurons to fire, might be replaced by more precise interventions—there have already been experimental attempts to stimulate specific brain regions to treat intractable depression (Mayberg et al., 2005).

Psychotherapy and the Future

It is ironic that psychiatry has adopted the principles of evidence-based medicine but applies those principles mainly to biological therapies and ignores the vast body of evidence showing that psychotherapy helps almost every kind of problem psychiatrists see. Patients are paying the price for this shortsightedness. Sadly, the main reason that psychother-apy is being ignored is financial. In a fee-for-service system, spending more time with each patient means psychiatrists see fewer patients. If physicians were remunerated differently, this would not be the case. Still, psychiatrists, no matter how strapped they are for time, can provide brief evidence-based psychotherapy.

Another reason psychotherapy is ignored is that drugs are believed to be more effective than talk. Psychiatrists still pay lip service to talk therapy, but their prescription pads speak louder than their words. Even psychiatrists who are convinced of the value of psychotherapy are in a position to provide only a fraction of the services patients need. They should be referring patients for psychotherapy—much as orthopedic surgeons routinely refer patients to physiotherapy. They can support psychologists and other mental health professionals who provide these services. (While longer treatment is not evidence-based and should be carried out only rarely, it is at least supportive for many people in distress.) Although not every patient will benefit from formal psychotherapy, this method needs to be tried, even with the most severely ill patients.

The Future Role of Psychiatrists

Everyone agrees that the current mental health care system is not working and that patients lack access to care. But beyond changes to the system (which are outside the scope of this book), psychiatrists in the future will have to practice differently than they currently do. They are highly trained specialists who should treat only the sickest patients. To treat the patients who need the most care, psychiatrists cannot continue working alone in offices and treating patients who could just as easily be managed by non-medical therapists. However, psychiatrists should continue to play a role in the treatment of less sick people by offering consultation, triage, and referral to appropriate services.

I work in an evaluation and consultation clinic attached to a teaching hospital. Every so often, I see patients who have been seen for many years by psychiatrists in private practice. When these physicians retired or moved away, I found virtually without exception that these patients easily could have been managed instead by a family doctor. Perhaps these psychiatrists felt more comfortable seeing old patients with familiar problems than new patients with unfamiliar problems.

Ironically, the DSM system provided psychiatrists with an excuse to see patients with less severe problems. By diagnosing almost every psychological problem as a mental illness, the DSM system brings the human condition itself within the scope of psychiatry. Even psychoanalysts point out (correctly) that they are seeing people with DSM diagnoses. The failure to make a distinction between a mental illness like major depression and normal unhappiness has real consequences for service delivery. It encourages psychiatrists to continue abandoning the severely mentally ill by concentrating on patients with milder symptoms who are not all that dysfunctional.

The idea that psychiatrists should treat the sickest patients does not invalidate in any way the suffering caused by less severe symptoms. Whether or not these problems qualify as true illnesses, many disorders listed in DSM are associated with a real burden and a real impact on functioning. Someone needs to help people with these problems, even if that turns out not to be psychiatrists. The model that best addresses the problem is one in which psychiatrists do what only *they* can do, and stop competing with other professionals, instead supporting other professionals to do what *they* do best. Let us look at how this might work out in practice.

Medicine is moving toward a system where the first line of treatment for all patients is to see family doctors. This procedure avoids the fragmentation of care that occurs when several specialists are involved. There is no reason that most patients with common mental health problems such as anxiety or depression cannot be treated by a family doctor (or by a nurse practitioner). In this system, only patients who family doctors cannot manage or who have already failed a first course of treatment would be referred to psychiatrists. But we have to restructure the primary care system to prevent doctor's offices from becoming factories where everyone gets seen for five minutes and is then shown the door.

Psychiatrists' skills in diagnosis are often needed to evaluate patients. We can pick up a missed psychosis or melancholia. We can also reassure our consultees when symptoms give no cause for alarm.

Psychiatrists are experts in psychopharmacology. But patients need that expertise only when simpler treatments fail to help. And many patients with severe mental disorders (such as schizophrenia and bipolar illness) reach a stable state in which they may need nothing more than renewals of the same dose of medication. There is no reason that these chronic patients should see a psychiatrist, except for an occasional consultation.

To make this "shared care" system work, psychiatrists have to work closely with other professionals and avoid isolating themselves in offices. They need to be readily available to consult with and support family doctors and other caregivers—by phone, in person, or through video-conferencing. The same structure could be applied to sharing the care of patients with psychologists. The implication is that psychiatrists would treat fewer patients directly and would spend much more time (perhaps as much as half their time) as consultants. Again, this system requires psychiatrists to work in groups and to be part of multidisciplinary teams. This is the kind of practice that belongs in clinics and hospitals, although it is not compatible with a private office.

Economics and Psychiatry

Most of my colleagues went into psychiatry out of idealism. But as people become successful, they can begin to feel entitled. This has happened, to some degree or other, to most of the psychiatrists I have known. The problem is that we can maximize their incomes in many ways but only at the expense of providing the services and skills that society needs.

Of course, psychiatrists are no better or worse than anyone else. Human nature being what it is, people will always find rationalizations for making more money. The problem is the system, and the answer lies in developing a different financial structure. We need to make psychiatry less sensitive to economic forces and more responsive to public health. We need a medical care system that rewards idealism and service.

I would like academics and researchers to be role models for this change. Recent disclosures about "consultancies" have led the National Institute for Mental Health to establish rules preventing its full-time researchers from receiving almost any outside income. This rule should be applied at every university. Professors should not be "for sale."

In clinical practice, a single-payer system would provide psychiatrists with a secure income, while the replacement of solo practice with teamwork would remove the temptation for psychiatrists to cultivate a practice of wealthy patients. The one thing that is least likely to change is that court testimony pays very well. But this kind of work will always constitute a small portion of psychiatric practice.

Obstacles to Change

There are several obstacles to implementing these changes in the practice of psychiatry. The first is medical autonomy. The concept of a physician as an independent practitioner remains a powerful tradition in U.S. medicine—even as it becomes obsolete. As shown by the United States' failure to develop any national health care system, culture and values have produced ferocious resistance to any change in how physicians work or how they are paid—often supported by the very public that suffers from lack of access to care.

The U.S. health care system is unique. The rest of the world has publicly funded universal health care systems, although in most other nations, patients dissatisfied with the public sector can pay for a better quality in the private sector. That kind of system retains autonomy for the patient and the physician but ensures at least a minimal standard of care for all. The American Psychiatric Association has a mandate to protect its members' autonomy and would oppose the kind of changes I am suggesting. Yet everyone is accountable to someone, and psychiatrists are no different. We should be public servants, not entrepreneurs.

The second obstacle to change is money. Psychiatrists are afraid of losing income. This raises the question of whether or not current methods of financial remuneration for physicians are ideal for patients receiving medical treatment. A fee-for-service model encourages quantity of services, but not necessarily quality. It also fails entirely to discriminate between patients who need the services of psychiatrists and those who do not.

If the economics of medicine is working against the rationalization of care, we need a new model that rewards physicians who look after sick people. A different system need not be excessively onerous. We already shape physician behavior in a number of ways—for example, by requiring continuing medical education and by encouraging evidence-based practice. And every psychiatrist is angry about Managed Care. We need a medical system that reinforces good practice without requiring financial sacrifice.

The third obstacle lies in human resources. There are not enough physicians in primary care settings to implement the changes I propose in this book, because there is a chronic shortage of medical students choosing family medicine. If family medicine paid better, more physicians might go into it. For my plan to work, patients will need to rely on these types of physicians to help them with less severe mental disorders, and psychiatrists will need these physicians to help support them. But without a proper support network, psychiatrists will be stuck in the same situation they are in today—helping everyone with a DSM diagnosis largely by doling out a drug prescription. Moreover, while we have enough psychologists to provide a high standard of care to the population, their services cost money, which neither insurers nor governments are keen to spend.

Behind these problems with limitations in resources lies the stigma of mental illness. The public would not tolerate such a level of care for non-psychiatric illness. Mental health services are chronically unfunded.

When psychiatric benefits are cut, patients do not go out into the street and demonstrate. Imagine what would happen if governments and insurance companies stopped paying for renal dialysis or chemotherapy on the grounds that such treatments are expensive.

Psychiatrists are not listened to when they complain about these problems; they are seen as merely defending their own interests. Organizations like the National Association for Mental Illness are in a better position to raise awareness about mental illness and to lobby for available treatment. And whenever celebrities (such as Brooke Shields) open up about a successful experience with psychiatry, offering themselves as a "poster child," all mental health professions gain credibility. To improve public support for the treatment of mental illness, psychiatrists need to spend time raising public awareness about the problem and reducing the stigma.

Psychiatry in 2050

Futurology can be comical—especially in retrospect. Even Jules Verne, who predicted the future with some accuracy, failed to anticipate the motorcar, imagining a 20th-century world still dominated by horsepower. As a child, I remember experts prognosticating in 1950 about what the next half century might bring. Most of their ideas were extensions of developments in the previous 50 years—such as ever more rapid transportation. Nobody anticipated that the most important technological development of the coming decades would be in communications and that the computer would change the world.

The distinguished forensic psychiatrist Paul Applebaum notes how often psychiatry has greeted false dawns, in which the answers to the mystery of mental illness have seemed to be forthcoming (Hobson & Leonard, 2001; Applebaum, 2004). Each of these periods—the heyday of psychoanalysis, the promise of community psychiatry, and the hegemony of biological psychiatry—has turned out to depend more on fads than on facts. The outcome has often been disappointment and disillusionment. We should be humble about how long it will take to find answers to difficult questions.

With these caveats in mind, I would nevertheless like to offer some educated guesses about what psychiatry will look like in the next 40 or so years.

- Psychiatrists will know more about the causes of major mental illnesses than they do today, and they will be able to directly measure the process of illness as it affects the brain.
- These advances will lead to a completely different diagnostic system based on the process of disease and not just on symptoms.
- These advances will also lead to treatment methods that are more precise. However, cures for the severest mental illnesses will remain a long way off.
- Psychotherapy will remain part of psychiatric practice but will consist of evidence-based and briefer treatments.
- Psychiatrists will devote most of their clinical time to the sickest patients and to the most difficult cases.
- Psychiatrists will spend more time on consultation and shared care. Fewer will work alone in offices, and the majority will practice in clinics and hospitals.
- Psychiatrists will earn most of their income from salaried employment or pooled funds, releasing them from economic motives that lead them away from their mission.

The Mission of Psychiatry

I look forward to a psychiatry that is neither brainless nor mindless but focuses on what is true and on what helps patients. The most important responsibility of psychiatrists is to care for the large number of people with mental illnesses, many of whom are currently receiving inadequate treatment. This mission requires serious changes in the pattern of service delivery. It also requires an ideological shift, both for health planners and for practitioners.

Research will continue to influence the future of psychiatry. As science develops, and as the mind and the brain are better understood, new methods of treatment will emerge. However, this does not mean that psychiatrists of the future must continue to focus exclusively on drug treatment. The commitment of psychiatry should be to science, and science tells us that both biological and psychological interventions are, each in their own way, prescriptions that can heal the mind.

Endnotes

Introduction

1. "Mindless" and "brainless," as turns of phrase, were actually first used by the Cornell University psychiatrist Robert Michels in a debate at the American Psychiatric Association meeting in Toronto in 1982 and published in Klerman et al., 1984.

Chapter 1

1. http://www.thinkexist.com/quotes/isaac_newton, accessed July 25, 2006.

Chapter 3

1. This manual was also published in 1952, 1968, 1980, 1987, and 1994.

Chapter 5

1. www.naminh.org/action-famous-people.php, accessed December 20, 2006.

Chapter 6

1. imagesoftheself.com/adhd_teacherParent_quest.pdf, accessed December 20, 2006.

Chapter 7

1. For a systematic approach to how psychiatry fits into the history of medicine, there is no better book than Shorter, 1997.
2. www.cochrane.org, accessed December 20, 2006.
3. http://www.psych.org/psych_pract/treatg/pg/prac_guide.cfm, accessed December 20, 2006.

Chapter 8

1. Much of the information about psychiatric drugs in this chapter can be found in standard textbooks (e.g., Sadock, Kaplan, & Sadock, 2004). Mental health professionals will probably be familiar with many points I make. For a detailed review of earlier research, see Bloom & Kupfer, 1995; for more recent findings see Schatzberg & Nemeroff, 2004.
2. http://www.psych.org/psych_pract/treatg/pg/MDD2e_05-15-06.pdf, accessed December 20, 2006.

Chapter 9

1. Much of this section is discussed in greater detail in my previous book; see Paris, 2006a.

Chapter 10

1. The 1998 survey was published in three parts: Marcus, Suarez, Tanielian, & Pincus, 2001; Suarez, Marcus, Tanielian, & Pincus, 2001; Tanielian, Marcus, Suarez, & Pincus, 2001; Scully & Wilk, 2003. Data from the 2002 survey were presented in more detail at a conference: see Regier, 2003.
2. President's New Freedom Report on Mental Health, 2003, www.mental healthcommission.gov/reports/FinalReport/downloads/ExecSummary.pdf, accessed December 20, 2006.

Chapter 12

1. For a review of this subject, see Gutheil, 1998.
2. www.forensic-serotonin.com, accessed December 20, 2006; www.courttv
   .com/trials/sharpe/112701_ctv.html, accessed December 20, 2006.
3. A good standard text about the issues discussed in this section is Simon &
   Gold, 2004.
4. www.law.umkc.edu/faculty/projects/ftrials/hinckley/hinckleytrial.html, accessed
   December 20, 2006.
5. For a good textbook reviewing the issues discussed in this section, see Eaton,
   2000.

References

Abrams, R., & Taylor, M. A. (1981). Importance of schizophrenic symptoms in the diagnosis of mania. *American Journal of Psychiatry, 138*, 658–661.

Achenbach, T. M., & McConaughy, S. H. (1997). *Empirically based assessment of child and adolescent psychopathology: Practical applications* (2nd ed.). Thousand Oaks, CA: Sage Publications.

Akiskal, H. S. (2002). The bipolar spectrum: The shaping of a new paradigm in psychiatry. *Current Psychiatry Reports, 4*, 1–3.

Akiskal, H. S., & McKinney, W. T. Jr. (1973). Depressive disorders: Toward a unified hypothesis. *Science, 182*, 20–29.

Alberts, D. S., Martinez, M. E., Roe, D. J., Guillen-Rodriguez, J. M., Marshall, J. R., van Leeuwen, J. B., et al. (2000). Lack of effect of a high-fiber cereal supplement on the recurrence of colorectal adenomas. *The New England Journal of Medicine, 342*, 1156–1162.

Alexander, F., & French, T. (1946). *Psychoanalytic therapy*. New York: Ronald Press.

American Psychiatric Association. (1952). *Diagnostic and statistical manual of mental disorders*. Washington, DC: American Psychiatric Press.

American Psychiatric Association. (1968). *Diagnostic and statistical manual of mental disorders* (2nd ed.). Washington, DC: American Psychiatric Press.

American Psychiatric Association. (1980). *Diagnostic and statistical manual of mental disorders* (3rd ed.). Washington, DC: American Psychiatric Press.

American Psychiatric Association. (1987). *Diagnostic and statistical manual of mental disorders, Revised* (3rd ed.). Washington, DC: American Psychiatric Press.

American Psychiatric Association. (1994). *Diagnostic and statistical manual of mental disorders* (4th ed.). Washington, DC: American Psychiatric Press.

American Psychiatric Association. (2000). *Diagnostic and statistical manual of mental disorders, Text revision* (4th ed.). Washington, DC: American Psychiatric Press.

American Psychiatric Association. (2002). *Practice guideline for the treatment of patients with major depressive disorder* (2nd ed.). Washington, DC: American Psychiatric Press.

Andreasen, N. C. (2001). *Brave new brain: Conquering mental illness in the era of the genome.* New York: Oxford University Press.

Angell, M. (2005). *The truth about the drug companies.* New York: Random House.

Angst, J., & Gamma, A. (2002). A new bipolar spectrum concept: a brief review. *Bipolar Disorders, 4,* 11–14.

Applebaum, P. (2004). Foreword. In J. Radden (Ed.), *The philosophy of psychiatry* (pp. vii–ix). New York: Oxford University Press.

Asarnow, R. F., Nuechterlein, K. H., Fogelson, D., Subotnik, K. L., Payne, D. A., Russell, A. T., et al. (2001). Schizophrenia and schizophrenia-spectrum personality disorders in the first-degree relatives of children with schizophrenia: the UCLA family study. *Archives of General Psychiatry, 58,* 581–588.

Avenell, A., Gillespie, W. J., Gillespie, L. D., & O'Connell, D. L. (2005). Vitamin D and vitamin D analogues for preventing fractures associated with involutional and post-menopausal osteoporosis. *Cochrane database of dystematic reviews,* Issue 3. Art. No.: CD000227. DOI: 10.1002/14651858.CD000227. pub2.

Avorn, J. (2004). *Powerful medicines.* New York: Random House.

Baghai, T. C., Moller, H. J., & Rupprecht, R. (2006). Recent progress in pharmacological and non-pharmacological treatment options of major depression. *Current Pharmaceutical Design, 12(4),* 503–515.

Barbui, C., & Hotopf, M. (2001). Amitriptyline v. the rest: still the leading antidepressant after 40 years of randomised controlled trials. *British Journal of Psychiatry, 178,* 129–144.

Baxter, L. R., Schwartz, J. M., & Bergman, K. S. (1992). Caudate glucose metabolic rate changes with both drug and behavior therapy for obsessive-compulsive disorder. *Archives of General Psychiatry, 49,* 618–689.

Beck, A. T. (1986). *Cognitive therapy and the emotional disorders.* New York: Basic.

Beckermann, A., Flohr, H., & Kim, J. (Eds.). (1992). *Emergence or reduction? Essays on the prospects of nonreductive physicalism.* Berlin: Walter de Gruyter.

Bender, D. A. (2002). Daily doses of multivitamin tablets. *British Medical Journal, 325,* 173–174.

Berrettini, W. H. (2005). Genetic bases for endophenotypes in psychiatric disorders. *Dialogues in Clinical Neuroscience, 7,* 95–101.

Biederman, J. (2005). Attention-deficit/hyperactivity disorder: A selective overview. *Biological Psychiatry, 57,* 1215–1220.

Birmaher, B., Axelson, D., Strober, M., Gill, M. K., Valeri, S., Chiappetta, L., Ryan, N., Leonard, H., Hunt, J., Iyengar, S., & Keller, M. (2006). Clinical course of children and adolescents with bipolar spectrum disorders. *Archives of General Psychiatry, 63,* 175–183.

Black, D. W. (1999). *Bad boys, bad men: Confronting antisocial personality.* New York: Oxford University Press.

Bleuler, E. (1950). *Dementia praecox, or the group of schizophrenias.* New York: International Universities Press.

Bliss, M. (2002). *William Osler: A life in medicine.* Toronto, ON: University of Toronto Press.

Bloom, F. E., & Kupfer, D. J. (Eds.). (1995). *Psychopharmacology: The fourth generation of progress* (4th ed.). New York: Raven Press.

Borus, J. F., & Olendzki, M. C. (1985). The offset effect of mental health treatment on ambulatory medical care utilization and charges. *Archives of General Psychiatry, 42,* 573–580.

Bowden, C. L., & Karren, N. U. (2006). Anticonvulsants in bipolar disorder. *Australian & New Zealand Journal of Psychiatry, 40,* 386–393.

Bowlby, J. (1969–1980). *Attachment and loss* (Vols. 1–3). London, UK: Hogarth Press.

Braff, D. L., Freedman, R., Schork, N. J., & Gottesman I. I. (2007). Deconstructing schizophrenia: An overview of the use of endophenotypes in order to understand a complex disorder. *Schizophrenia Bulletin, 33,* 21–32.

Breggin, P. (1994). *Toxic psychiatry: Why therapy, empathy and love must replace the drugs, electroshock, and biochemical theories of the "new psychiatry."* New York, St. Martin's Press.

Brestan, E. V., & Eyberg, S. M. (1998). Effective psychosocial treatments of conduct-disordered children and adolescents. *Journal of Clinical Child Psychology, 27,* 138–145.

Butler, A. C., Chapman, J. E., Forman, E. M., & Beck, A. T. (2006). The empirical status of cognitive-behavioral therapy: A review of meta-analyses. *Clinical Psychology Review, 26,* 17–31.

Cantor-Graae, E. (2007). The contribution of social factors to the development of schizophrenia. *Canadian Journal of Psychiatry, 52,* 277–286.

Carey, B. (2005a, June 18). Snake phobias, moodiness and a battle in psychiatry. Retrieved December 20, 2006, from the *New York Times.*

Carey, B. (2005b, June 12). Who's mentally ill? Deciding is often all in the mind. *New York Times.*

Carver C. S., & Miller, C. J. (2006). Relations of serotonin function to personality: Current views and a key methodological issue. *Psychiatry Research, 144,* 1–15.

Casacalenda, N., & Boulanger, J. P. (1998). Pharmacologic treatments effective in both generalized anxiety disorder and major depressive disorder: Clinical and theoretical implications. *Canadian Journal of Psychiatry, 43,* 722–730.

Casacalenda, N., Perry, J. C., & Looper, K. (2002). Remission in major depressive disorder: A comparison of pharmacotherapy, psychotherapy, and control conditions. *American Journal of Psychiatry, 159,* 1354–1360.

Caspi, A., McClay, J., Moffitt, T. E., Mill, J., Martin, J., Craig, I. W., et al. (2002). Role of genotype in the cycle of violence in maltreated children. *Science, 297,* 851–854.

Caspi, A., Sugden, K., Moffitt, T. E., Taylor, A., Craig, I. W., Harrington, H., et al. (2003). Influence of life stress on depression: Moderation by a polymorphism in the 5–HTT gene. *Science, 301,* 386–389.

Cassidy, J., & Shaver, P. R. (Eds.). (1999). *Handbook of attachment: Theory, research and clinical aspects.* New York: Guilford Press.

Churchland, P. (1995). *The engine of reason, the seat of the soul: A philosophical journey into the brain.* Cambridge: MIT Press.

Cooper, J. E., Kendell, R. E., & Gurland, B. J. (1972). *Psychiatric diagnosis in New York and London.* London: Oxford University Press.

Coyle, J. T. (2006). Glutamate and schizophrenia: Beyond the dopamine hypothesis. *Cellular & Molecular Neurobiology, 26,* 365–384.

Crits-Christoph, P., & Barber, J. (Eds.). (1991). *Handbook of short-term dynamic psychotherapy.* New York: Basic Books.

Dale, K. M., Coleman, C. I., Henyan, N. N., Kluger, J., & White, C. M. (2006). Statins and cancer risk: A meta-analysis. *JAMA: The Journal of the American Medical Association, 295,* 74–80.

Dawes, R. M. (1994). *House of cards: Psychology and psychotherapy built on myth.* New York: Free Press.

Delate, T., Gelenberg, A. J., Simmons, V. A., & Motheral, B. R. (2004). Trends in the use of antidepressants in a national sample of commercially insured pediatric patients, 1998 to 2002. *Psychiatric Services, 55,* 387–391.

Dennett, D. (1991). *Consciousness explained.* Boston: Back Bay.

Devilly, G. J., & Spence, S. H. (1999). The relative efficacy and treatment distress of EMDR and a cognitive-behavior trauma treatment protocol in the amelioration of posttraumatic stress disorder. *Journal of Anxiety Disorders, 13,* 131–157.

Dewan, M. J., Steenbarger, B. N., & Greenberg, R. P. (Eds.). (2004). *The art and science of brief psychotherapies: A practitioner's guide.* Washington, DC: American Psychiatric Publishing.

Doidge, N., Simon, B., Brauer, L., Grant, D. C., First, M., Brunshaw, J., et al. (2002a). Psychoanalytic patients in the U.S., Canada, and Australia: I. DSM-III-R disorders, indications, previous treatment, medications, and length of treatment. *Journal of the American Psychoanalytic Association, 50,* 575–614.

Doidge, N., Simon, B., Lancee, W. J., First, M., Brunshaw, J., Brauer, L., et al. (2002b). Psychoanalytic patients in the U.S., Canada, and Australia: II. A DSM-III-R validation study. *Journal of the American Psychoanalytic Association, 50,* 615–627.

Dolnick, E. (1998). *Madness on the couch.* New York: Simon and Schuster.

Downs, L. L. (2002). PMS, psychosis and culpability: Sound or misguided defense? *Journal of Forensic Science, 47,* 1083–1089.

Doyle, A. E., Willcutt, E. G., Seidman, L. J., Biederman, J., Chouinard, V. A., Silva, J., et al. (2005). Attention-deficit/hyperactivity disorder endophenotypes. *Biological Psychiatry, 57,* 1324–1335.

Duffy, A. (2007). Does bipolar disorder exist in children? A selected review. *Canadian Journal of Psychiatry, 52*(7), 409–417

Duncan, B. L. (2002). The legacy of Saul Rosenzweig: The profundity of the dodo bird. *Journal of Psychotherapy Integration, 12,* 32–57.

Eaton, W. W. (2000). *The sociology of mental disorders* (3rd ed.). New York: Greenwood.

Eisenberg, L. (1986). Mindlessness and brainlessness in psychiatry. *British Journal of Psychiatry, 148,* 497–508.

Eisenberg, L. (1995). The social construction of the human brain. *American Journal of Psychiatry, 152,* 1563–1575.

Eisenberg, L. (1997). Past, present, and future of psychiatry: Personal reflections. *Canadian Journal of Psychiatry, 42,* 705–713.

Eisenberg, L. (2000). Is psychiatry more mindful or brainier than it was a decade ago? *British Journal of Psychiatry, 176,* 1–5.

Eisenberg, L. (2004). Social psychiatry and the human genome: Contextualising heritability. *British Journal of Psychiatry, 184,* 101–103.

Elkin, I., Shea, T., Watkins, J. T., & Imber, S. D. (1989). National Institute of Mental Health Treatment of Depression Collaborative Research Program: General effectiveness of treatments, *Archives of General Psychiatry, 46,* 971–982.

Emsley, R., & Oosthuizen, P. (2003). The new and evolving pharmacotherapy of schizophrenia. *Psychiatric Clinics of North America, 26,* 141–163.

Engel, G. L. (1980). The clinical application of the biopsychosocial model. *The American Journal of Psychiatry, 137,* 535–544.

Evidence-Based Medicine Working Group. (1992). Evidence-based medicine: A new approach to teaching the practice of medicine. *JAMA: The Journal of the American Medical Association, 268,* 2420–2425.

Eysenck, H. (1952). The effects of psychotherapy: An evaluation. *Journal of Consulting Psychology, 16,* 319–324.

Eysenck, H. J. (1973). *Handbook of Abnormal Psychology.* London: Pitman.

Faulkner, L. R., & Goldman, C. R. (1997). Estimating psychiatric manpower requirements based on patients' needs. *Psychiatric Services, 48,* 666–670.

Fava, M., & Rankin, M. (2002). Sexual functioning and SSRIs. *Journal of Clinical Psychiatry, 63*(Suppl. 5), 13–16.

Fawcett, I., Stein, D. J., & Jobson, K. O. (Eds.). (1999). *Textbook of treatment algorithms in psychopharmacology.* New York: John Wiley.

Feil, E., Welch, G., & Fisher, E. (1993). Why estimates of physician supply and requirements disagree. *JAMA: The Journal of the American Medical Association, 269,* 2659–2663.

First, M. B. (2005). Mutually exclusive versus co-occurring diagnostic categories: The challenge of diagnostic comorbidity. *Psychopathology, 38,* 206–210.

First, M. B., Spitzer, R. L., Gibbon, M., & Williams, J. B. W. (1997a). *Structured clinical interview for DSM-IV Axis I disorders (SCID-I), Clinician Version.* Washington, DC: American Psychiatric Press.

First, M. B., Spitzer, R. L., Gibbon, M., & Williams, J. B. W. (1997b). *Structured clinical interview for DSM-IV Axis II disorders (SCID-II).* Washington, DC: American Psychiatric Press.

First, M. B., & Zimmerman, M. (2006). Including laboratory tests in DSM-V diagnostic criteria. *American Journal of Psychiatry, 163,* 2041–2042.

Fisher, B., Jeong, J.-H., Anderson, S., Bryant, J., Fisher, E. R., & Wolmark, N. (2002). Twenty-five-year follow-up of a randomized trial comparing radical mastectomy, total mastectomy, and total mastectomy followed by irradiation. *New England Journal of Medicine, 347,* 567–575.

Fisher, S., & Greenberg, R. (1996). *Freud scientifically reappraised: Testing the theories and therapy.* New York: Wiley & Sons.

Flint, J., & Munafo, M. R. (2007). The endophenotype concept in psychiatric genetics. *Psychological Medicine, 37,* 163–180.

Foa, E. B., Cahill, S. P., Boscarino, J. A., Hobfoll, S. E., Lahad, M., McNally, R. J., et al. (2005). Social, psychological, and psychiatric interventions following terrorist attacks: Recommendations for practice and research. *Neuropsychopharmacology, 30,* 1806–1817.

Foa, E. B., Rothbaum, B. O., & Furr, J. M. (2003). Augmenting exposure therapy with other CBT procedures. *Psychiatric Annals, 33,* 47–53.

Frank, J. D., & Frank, J. B. (1991). *Persuasion and healing* (3rd ed.). Baltimore: Johns Hopkins.

Freud, S. (1957). The aetiology of hysteria. In J. Strachey (Ed. & Trans.), *The standard edition of the complete psychological works of Sigmund Freud* (Vol. 3, pp. 191–224). London: Hogarth Press. (Original work published 1896).

Freud, S. (1958). A general introduction to psychoanalysis. In J. Strachey (Ed. & Trans.), *The standard edition of the complete psychological works of Sigmund Freud* (Vol. 15 & 16). London: Hogarth Press. (Original work published 1916).

Freud, S. (1964). Analysis terminable and interminable. In J. Strachey (Ed. & Trans.), *The standard edition of the complete psychological works of Sigmund Freud* (Vol. 23, pp. 216–254). London: Hogarth Press. (Original work published 1937).

Gabbard, G. O. (2004). *Long–term psychodynamic psychotherapy: A basic text.* Washington, DC: American Psychiatric Press.

Gabbard, G. O. (2000). A neurobiologically informed perspective on psychotherapy. *The British Journal of Psychiatry, 177,* 117–122.

Gabbard, G. O., Lazar, S. G., Hornberger, J., & Speigel, D. (1997). The economic impact of psychotherapy: A review. *American Journal of Psychiatry, 154,* 147–155.

Gansler, D. A., Fucetola, R., Krengel, M., Stetson, S., Zimering, R., & Makary, C. (1998). Are there cognitive subtypes in adult attention deficit/hyperactivity disorder? *Journal of Nervous & Mental Disease, 186,* 776–781.

Ghaemi, S. N., Ko, J. Y., & Goodwin, F. K. (2002). "Cade's disease" and beyond: misdiagnosis, antidepressant use, and a proposed definition for bipolar spectrum disorder. *Canadian Journal of Psychiatry, 47,* 125–134.

Ghaemi, S. N., Soldani, F., & Hsu, D. J. (2003). Evidence–based pharmacotherapy of bipolar disorder. *International Journal of Neuropsychopharmacology, 6,* 303–308.

Goldberg, D. (2006). The aetiology of depression. *Psychological Medicine, 36,* 1341–1347.

Goldberg, D., & Goodyer, I. (2005). *The origins and course of common mental disorders.* London: Taylor and Francis.

Goode, E. (2000, January 11). Scientist at work: Aaron T. Beck; Pragmatist embodies his no-nonsense therapy. Retrieved December 20, 2006, from the *New York Times* Web site: http://nytimes.com.

Goodwin, F. K., Fireman, B., Simon, G. E., Hunkeler, E. M., Lee, J., & Revicki, D. (2003). Suicide risk in bipolar disorder during treatment with lithium and divalproex. *JAMA: The Journal of the American Medical Association, 290,* 1467–1473.

Goodwin, F. K., & Ghaemi, N. (2003). The course of bipolar disorder and the nature of agitated depression. *American Journal of Psychiatry, 160,* 2077–2079.

Goodwin, F. K., & Jamison, K. (2007): Manic-depressive illness: Bipolar disorder and recurrent depression (2nd ed.). New York: Oxford University Press.

Gottman, J. M., Driver, J., & Tabares, A. (2002). Building the sound marital house: An empirically derived couple therapy. In A. S. Gurman & N. S. Jacobson (Eds.), *Clinical handbook of couple therapy* (3rd ed., pp. 373–399). New York: Guilford Press.

Grant, B. F., Hasin, D. S., Stinson, F. S., Dawson, D. A., Chou, S. P., Ruan, W. J., et al. (2004). Prevalence, correlates, and disability of personality disorders in the United States: Results from the national epidemiologic survey on alcohol and related conditions. *Journal of Clinical Psychiatry, 65,* 948–958.

Grigoraidis, V. (2004). Are you bipolar? *New York Magazine.* March 1.

Grinfeld, M. J. (1999). Recovered memory lawsuit sparks litigation. *Psychiatric Times, 16,* 12.

Grinker, R. R. (1964). Psychiatry rushes madly in all directions. *Archives of General Psychiatry, 10,* 228–237.

Groopman, J. (2007). *How doctors think.* Boston: Houghton Mifflin.

Grunbaum, A. (1984). *The foundations of psychoanalysis.* Berkeley: University of California Press.

Gunderson, J. G. (2001). *Borderline personality disorder: A clinical guide.* Washington, DC: American Psychiatric Press.

Gutheil, T. G. (1998). *The psychiatrist as expert witness.* Washington, DC: American Psychiatric Press.

Hale, R. (1995). *The rise and crisis of psychoanalysis in the United States.* New York: Oxford University Press.

Halleck, S. L. (1990). Dissociative phenomena and the question of responsibility. *International Journal of Clinical and Experimental Hypnosis, 38*(4), 298–314.

Hare, R. (1999). *Without conscience: The disturbing world of the psychopaths among us.* New York: Guilford Press.

Harris, J. R. (1998). *The nurture assumption.* New York: Free Press.

Healy, D. (1999). *The antidepressant era.* Cambridge, MA: Harvard University Press.

Helzer, J. E., & Canino, G. J. (Eds.). (1992). Alcoholism in North America, Europe, and Asia. New York: Oxford University Press.

Henry, C., Mitropoulou, V., New, A. S., Koenigsberg, H. W., Silverman, J., & Siever, L. J. (2001). Affective instability and impulsivity in borderline personality and bipolar II disorders: similarities and differences. *Journal of Psychiatric Research, 35,* 307–312.

Herman, J. (1992). *Trauma and recovery*. New York: Basic.

Hobson, J. A., Leonard, J. A. (2001). Out of Its Mind: Psychiatry in Crisis, a Call for Reform. New York: Basic.

Hoch, P. H., Cattell, J. P., Strahl, M. D., & Penness, H. H. (1962). The course and outcome of pseudoneurotic schizophrenia. *American Journal of Psychiatry, 119*, 106–115.

Hodges, B., Rubin, A., Cooke, R. G., Parker, S., & Adlaf, E. (2006). Factors predicting practice location and outreach consultation among University of Toronto psychiatry graduates. *Canadian Journal of Psychiatry, 51*, 218–225.

Hodgins, S. (2001). The major mental disorders and crime: Stop debating and start treating and preventing. *International Journal of Law & Psychiatry, 24*, 427–446.

Hogarty, G. E., Schooler, N. R., & Baker, R. W. (1997). Efficacy versus effectiveness. *Psychiatric Services, 48*, 1107.

Hollingshead, A., & Redlich, F. (1958). *Social class and mental illness*. New York: Wiley.

Holmes, O. W. (1972). *The works of Oliver Wendell Holmes*. St. Clair Shores, MI: Scholarly Press. pp. 306–309.

Horwitz, A. V., & Wakefield, J. C. (2007). *The loss of sadness: How psychiatry transformed normal sorrow into depressive disorder*. New York: Oxford University Press.

Howard, K. I., Kopta, A. M., Krause, M. S., & Orlinsky, D. E. (1986). The dose-effect relationship to psychotherapy. *American Psychologist, 41*, 159–164.

Insel, T., & Quirion, R. (2005). Psychiatry as a clinical neuroscience discipline. *JAMA: The Journal of the American Medical Association, 294*, 2221–2224.

Insel, T. R., & Fenton, W. S. (2005). Psychiatric epidemiology: It's not just about counting anymore. *Archives of General Psychiatry, 62*, 590–592.

Iversen, L. (2006). Neurotransmitter transporters and their impact on the development of psychopharmacology. *British Journal of Pharmacology, 147* (Suppl. 1), S82–8.

Jablow, D. H. (2002). *Power beyond reason: The mental collapse of Lyndon Johnson*. Fort Lee, NJ: Barricade Books.

Jamison, K. R. (1993). *Touched with fire: Manic-depressive illness and the artistic temperament*. Simon and Schuster.

Janet, P. (1901). *The mental state of hystericals*. New York: Putnam and Sons. (Reprinted in 1977 by University Publications of America, Washington, DC).

Jensen, P. S., Martin, D., & Cantwell, D. P. (1997). Comorbidity in ADHD: Implications for research, practice, and DSM–V. *Journal of the American Academy of Child & Adolescent Psychiatry, 36*, 1065–1079.

Johnston, M. (1997): *Spectral evidence: The Ramona case: Incest, memory, and truth on trial in Napa Valley.* Boulder, CO: Westview Press.

Jones, A., Cork, C., & Chowdhury, U. (2006). Autistic spectrum disorders. 1: Presentation and assessment. *Community Practitioner, 79,* 97–98.

Jones, R. H. (2000). *Reductionism: Analysis and the fullness of reality.* Lewisburg, PA: Bucknell University Press.

Judd, L. L., Schettler, P. J., Akiskal, H. S., Maser, J., Coryell, W., Solomon, D., et al. (2003). Long-term symptomatic status of bipolar I vs. bipolar II disorders. *International Journal of Neuropsychopharmacology, 6,* 127–137.

Kates, N., Craven, M., Bishop, J., Clinton, T., Kraftcheck, D., LeClair, K., et al. (2006). Shared mental health care in Canada. *Canadian Journal of Psychiatry, 56*(Suppl. 1), 21–67.

Kazdin, A. E. (1996). *Conduct disorder in childhood and adolescence* (2nd ed.). Thousand Oaks, CA: Sage.

Keller, M. B. (2005). Issues in treatment-resistant depression. *Journal of Clinical Psychiatry, 66*(8), 5–12.

Kendler, K. S. (2006). Reflections on the relationship between psychiatric genetics and psychiatric nosology. *American Journal of Psychiatry, 163,* 1138–1146.

Kendler, K. S., Neale, M., & Kessler, R. (1995). The structure of the genetic and environmental risk factors for six major psychiatric disorders in women. *Archives of General Psychiatry, 52,* 470–474.

Kessler, R. C., Chiu, W. T., Demler, O., Merikangas, K. R., & Walters, E. E. (2005). Prevalence, severity, and comorbidity of 12-month DSM–IV disorders in the National Comorbidity Survey Replication. *Archives of General Psychiatry, 62,* 617–627.

Kessler, R. C., Coccaro, E. F., Fava, M., Jaeger, S., Jin, R., & Walter, E. (2006). The prevalence and correlates of *DSM-IV* Intermittent Explosive Disorder in the National Comorbidity Survey Replication. *Archives of General Psychiatry, 63,* 669–678.

Kessler, R. C., McGonagle, K. A., Zhao, S., Nelson, C. B., Hughes, M., Eshleman, S., Wittchen, H. U., Kendler, K. S. (1994). Lifetime and 12-month prevalence of DSM-III-R psychiatric disorders in the United States. Results from the National Comorbidity Survey. Arch Gen Psychiatry, *51*(1), 8–19.

Kessler, R. C., Merikangas, K. R., Berglund, P., Eaton, W. W., Koretz, D. S., & Walters, E. E. (2003). Mild disorders should not be eliminated from the DSM–V. *Archives of General Psychiatry, 60,* 1117–1122.

Kiesler, C. A., Cummings, N. A., & VandenBos, G. R. (1979). *Psychology and national health insurance: A sourcebook.* Washington, DC: American Psychological Association.

Klein, D. F. (1987). Anxiety reconceptualized: Gleaning from pharmacological dissection—early experience with imipramine and anxiety. *Modern Problems of Pharmacopsychiatry, 22*, 1–35.

Klein, D. N., & Santiago, N. J. (2003). Dysthymia and chronic depression: Introduction, classification, risk factors, and course. *Journal of Clinical Psychology, 59*, 807–816.

Klerman, G. L., DiMascio, A., Weissman, M. M., Prusoff, B., & Paykel, E. E. (1974). Treatment of depression by drugs and psychotherapy. *American Journal of Psychiatry, 131*, 186–191.

Klerman, G. L., Vaillant, G. E., Spitzer, R. L., & Michels, R. (1984). A debate on DSM-III. *American Journal of Psychiatry, 141(4)*, 539–553.

Kocsis, J. H. (2003). Pharmacotherapy for chronic depression. *Journal of Clinical Psychology, 59*, 885–892.

Kondro, W. (2002). Income–based health premium centrepiece of Kirby report. *Canadian Medical Association Journal, 167*, 1279.

Kraepelin, E. (1921). Manic-depressive insanity and paranoia (R. M. Barclay, Trans.). G. M. Robertson, Ed. Edinburgh: E. and S. Livingstone. (Original work published 1913).

Krakowski, M. (2003). Violence and serotonin: Influence of impulse control, affect regulation, and social functioning. *Journal of Neuropsychiatry & Clinical Neurosciences, 15*, 294–305.

Kramer, P. (1993). *Listening to Prozac*. New York: Viking.

Krueger, R. F. (1999). The structure of common mental disorders. *Archives of General Psychiatry, 56*, 921–926.

Kupfer, D. J., First, M. B., & Regier, D. A. (2002). *A research agenda for DSM-V*. Washington, DC: American Psychiatric Press.

Lambert, M. (2003). *Bergin and Garfield's Handbook of Psychotherapy and Behavior Change*. New York: Wiley.

Leung, A. K., & Lemay, J. F. (2003). Attention deficit hyperactivity disorder: An update. *Advances in Therapeutics, 20*, 305–318.

Lieberman, J. A., Stroup, T. S., McEvoy, J. P., Swartz, M. S., Rosenheck, R. A., Perkins, D. O., et al. (2005). Clinical antipsychotic trials of intervention effectiveness (CATIE) investigators: Effectiveness of antipsychotic drugs in patients with chronic schizophrenia. *New England Journal of Medicine, 353*, 1209–1223.

Linde, K., Mulrow, C. D., Berner, M., & Egger, M. (2005). St John's wort for depression. *Cochrane Database of Systematic Reviews*, Issue 2. Art. No.: CD000448. DOI: 10.1002/14651858. CD000448.pub2.

Linehan, M. M. (1993). *Dialectical behavioral therapy of borderline personality disorder*. New York: Guilford Press.

Livesley, W. J. (Ed.). (2001). *Handbook of personality disorders: Theory, research, and treatment.* New York: Guilford Press.

Lopez, A. D., Mathers, C. D., Ezzati, M., Jamison, D. T., & Murray, C. J. (2006). Global and regional burden of disease and risk factors, 2001: Systematic analysis of population health data. *Lancet, 367,* 1747–1757.

Lovejoy, D. W., Diefenbach, G. J., Licht, D. J., & Tolin, D. F. (2003). Tracking levels of psychiatric distress associated with the terrorist events of September 11, 2001: A review of the literature. *Journal of Insurance Medicine, 35,* 114–124.

Luborsky, E., & Luborsky, L. (2006). *Research and psychotherapy: The vital link.* Jason Aronson.

Luborsky, L., Singer, B., & Luborsky, L. (1975). Comparative studies of psychotherapy: Is it true that "everyone has won and all shall have prizes"? *Archives of General Psychiatry, 41,* 165–180.

Luhrmann, T. (2000). *Of two minds.* New York: Norton.

Malcolm, J. (1982). *Psychoanalysis: The impossible profession.* New York: Vintage.

Mandzia, J., & Black, S. E. (2001). Neuroimaging and behavior: Probing brain behavior relationships in the 21st century. *Current Neurology & Neuroscience Reports, 1,* 553–561.

March, J. S., Silva, S. G., Compton, S., Shapiro, M., Califf, R., & Krishnan, R. (2005). The case for practical clinical trials in psychiatry. *American Journal of Psychiatry, 162,* 836–846.

Marcus, S. C., Suarez, A. P., Tanielian, T. L., & Pincus, H. A. (2001). Datapoints: Trends in psychiatric practice, 1988–1998: I. Demographic characteristics of practicing psychiatrists. *Psychiatric Services, 52,* 732.

Martin, J. P. (2002). The integration of neurology, psychiatry, and neuroscience in the 21st century. *American Journal of Psychiatry, 159,* 695–704.

Maughan, B., Rowe, R., Messer, J., Goodman, R., & Meltzer, H. (2004). Conduct disorder and oppositional defiant disorder in a national sample: Developmental epidemiology. *Journal of Child Psychology & Psychiatry & Allied Disciplines, 45,* 609–621.

Mayberg, H. S., Lozano, A. M., Voon, V., McNeely, H. E., Seminowicz, D., Hamani, C., et al. (2005). Deep brain stimulation for treatment-resistant depression. *Neuron, 45,* 651–660.

Mazziotta, J. C. (2000). Imaging: Window on the brain. *Archives of Neurology, 57,* 1413–1421.

McFarlane, A. C. (1989). The aetiology of post-traumatic morbidity: Predisposing, precipitating, and perpetuating factors. *British Journal of Psychiatry, 154,* 221–228.

McGorry, P. D., & Singh, B. S., 1995. Schizophrenia: Risk and possibility. In B. Raphael and G. D. Burrows (Eds.), *Handbook of preventive psychiatry* (pp. 492–514). Amsterdam: Elsevier.

McInnis, M. G., Dick, D. M., Willour, V. L., Avramopoulos, D., MacKinnon, D. F., Simpson, S. G., et al. (2003). Genome-wide scan and conditional analysis in bipolar disorder: Evidence for genomic interaction in the National Institute of Mental Health genetics initiative bipolar pedigrees. *Biological Psychiatry, 54,* 1265–1273.

McNally, R. (2003). *Remembering trauma.* Cambridge, MA: Belknap, Harvard University Press.

McNally, R. J. (1999). Post-traumatic stress disorder. In T. Millon, P. Blaney, & R. Davis (Eds.), *Oxford textbook of psychopathology* (pp. 144–165). New York: Oxford University Press.

Meaney, M. J., & Szyf, M. (2005). Environmental programming of stress responses through DNA methylation: Life at the interface between a dynamic environment and a fixed genome. *Dialogues in Clinical Neuroscience, 7,* 103–123.

Mechanic, D., & Bilder, S. (2004). Treatment of people with mental illness: A decade-long perspective. *Health Affairs, 23,* 84–95.

Meehl, P. E. (1990). Toward an integrated theory of schizotaxia, schizotypy, and schizophrenia. *Journal of Personality Disorders, 4,* 1–99.

Mellman, L. A. (2006). How endangered is dynamic psychiatry in residency training? *Journal of the American Academy of Psychoanalysis & Dynamic Psychiatry, 34,* 127–133.

Meltzer, H. Y., Alphs, L., Green, A. I., Altamura, A. C., Anand, R., Bertoldi, A., et al. (2003). Clozapine treatment for suicidality in schizophrenia: International Suicide Prevention Trial (InterSePT). *Archives of General Psychiatry, 60,* 82–91.

Menninger, R. W., & Nemiah, J. C. (2000). *American psychiatry after World War II, 1944–1994.* Washington, DC: American Psychiatric Press.

Middleton, H., Shaw, I., & Feder, G. (2005). NICE guidelines for the management of depression. *British Medical Journal, 330,* 267–268.

Moffit, T. E. (2001). *Sex differences in antisocial behaviour: Conduct disorder, delinquency, and violence in the Dunedin longitudinal study.* New York: Cambridge University Press.

Moncrieff, J., Wessely, S., & Hardy, R. (2004). Active placebos versus antidepressants for depression. *Cochrane database of systematic reviews,* Issue 1. Art. No.: CD003012. DOI: 10.1002/14651858.CD003012.pub2.

Monroe, S. M., & Simons, A. D. (1991). Diathesis-stress theories in the context of life stress research. *Psychological Bulletin, 110,* 406–425.

Montejo, A. L., Llorca, G., Izquierdo, J. A., & Rico-Villademoros, F. (2001). Incidence of sexual dysfunction associated with antidepressant agents: Spanish working group for the study of psychotropic-related sexual dysfunction: A prospective multicenter study of 1022 outpatients. *Journal of Clinical Psychiatry, 62*(Suppl. 3), 10–21.

Morihisa, J. M. (Ed.). (2001). *Advances in brain imaging*. Washington, DC: American Psychiatric Press.

Murphy, H. B. M. (1982). *Comparative psychiatry*. New York: Springer.

Nemeroff, C. B., Kilts, C. D., & Berns, G. S. (1999). Functional brain imaging: Twenty-first century phrenology or psychobiological advance for the millennium? *American Journal of Psychiatry, 15,* 671–673.

Nestler, E. J., Hyman, S. E., & Malenka, R. C. (Eds.). (2001). *Molecular neuropharmacology: A foundation for clinical neuroscience*. New York: McGraw Hill.

Newcomer, J. W., & Haupt, D. W. (2006). The metabolic effects of antipsychotic medication. *Canadian Journal of Psychiatry, 51,* 480–491.

Newton-Howes, G., Tyrer, P., & Johnson, T. (2006). Personality disorder and the outcome of depression: Meta-analysis of published studies. *British Journal of Psychiatry, 188,* 13–20.

Niculescu, A. B., & Akiskal, H. S. (2001). Proposed endophenotypes of dysthymia: Evolutionary, clinical and pharmacogenomic considerations. *Molecular Psychiatry, 6,* 363–366.

Nigg, J. T. (2006). Temperament and developmental psychopathology. *Journal of Child Psychology & Psychiatry & Allied Disciplines, 47,* 395–422.

Nigg, J. T., & Casey, B. J. (2005). An integrative theory of attention-deficit/hyperactivity disorder based on the cognitive and affective neurosciences. *Development & Psychopathology, 17,* 785–806.

Nunes, E. V., & Levin, F. R. (2004). Treatment of depression in patients with alcohol or other drug dependence: A meta-analysis. *JAMA: The Journal of the American Medical Association, 291,* 1887–1896.

Olfson, M., Blanco, C., Liu, L., Moreno, C., & Laje, G. (2006). National trends in the outpatient treatment of children and adolescents with antipsychotic drugs. *Archives of General Psychiatry, 63,* 679–685.

Olfson, M., Marcus, S. C., Druss, B., Elinson, L., Tanielian, T., & Pincus, A. (2002). National trends in the outpatient treatment of depression. *JAMA: The Journal of the American Medical Association, 287,* 203–209.

Olsen, O., & Gøtzsche, P. C. *Screening for breast cancer with mammography*. Cochrane Database Syst Rev 2001;(4): CD001877. 4.

Osler, W. (1898). *The principles and practice of medicine*. New York: Appleton.

Paris, J. (1996). *Social factors in the personality disorders*. Cambridge, UK: Cambridge University Press.

Paris, J. (1999). *Nature and nurture in psychiatry: A predisposition-stress model*. Washington, DC: American Psychiatric Press.

Paris, J. (2000a). *Myths of childhood*. Philadelphia, PA: Brunner/Mazzel, 2000.

Paris, J. (2000b). Predispositions, personality traits, and post-traumatic stress disorder. *Harvard Review of Psychiatry, 8,* 175–183.

Paris, J. (2003). *Personality Disorders over Time*. Washington, DC: American Psychiatric Press.

Paris, J. (2005a). *The fall of an icon: Psychoanalysis and academic psychiatry*. Toronto, ON: University of Toronto Press.

Paris, J. (2005b). Recent advances in the treatment of borderline personality disorder. *Canadian Journal of Psychiatry, 50,* 435–441.

Paris, J. (2006a). *Half in love with death: Managing the chronically suicidal patient*. Mahwah, NJ: Laurence Erlbaum.

Paris, J. (2006b). Predicting and preventing suicide: Do we know enough to do either? *Harvard Review of Psychiatry, 14,* 233–240.

Paris, J., Gunderson, J. G., & Weinberg, I. (in 2007). The interface between borderline personality disorder and bipolar spectrum disorder. *Comprehensive Psychiatry, 48,* 145–154.

Parker, G. (2005a). Beyond major depression. *Psychological Medicine, 35,* 467–474.

Parker, G. (2005b). Melancholia. *American Journal of Psychiatry, 162,* 1066.

Parker, G., & Manicavasagar, V. (Eds.). (2005). *Modelling and managing the depressive disorders*. Cambridge, UK: Cambridge University Press.

Patten, S. B. (2006). Does almost everybody suffer from a bipolar disorder? *Canadian Journal of Psychiatry, 51,* 6–8.

Paulose-Ram, R., Safran, M. A., Jonas, B. S., Gu, Q., & Orwig, D. (2007). Trends in psychotropic medication use among US adults. *Pharmacoepidemiology and Drug Safety, 16(5),* 560–570.

Pepper, C. M., Klein, D. N., Anderson, R. L., Riso, L. P., Ouimette, P. C., & Lizardi, H. (1995). DSM-III-R Axis II comorbidity in dysthymia and major depression. *American Journal of Psychiatry, 152,* 239–247.

Petronis, A., Gottesman, I. I., Crow, T. J., DeLisi, L. E., Klar, A. J., Macciardi, F., McInnis, M. G., McMahon, F. J., Paterson, A. D., Skuse, D., & Sutherland, G. R. (2000). Psychiatric epigenetics: A new focus for the new century. *Molecular Psychiatry, 5,* 342–346.

Pinker, S. (1997). *How the mind works*. New York: Norton.

Piper, A., & Merskey, H. (2004a). The persistence of folly: A critical examination of dissociative identity disorder. Part I. The excesses of an improbable concept. *Canadian Journal of Psychiatry, 49,* 592–600.

Piper A., & Merskey, H. (2004b). The persistence of folly: Critical examination of dissociative identity disorder. Part II. The defence and decline of multiple personality or dissociative identity disorder. *Canadian Journal of Psychiatry, 49,* 678–683.

Pitkin, J., Rees, M. C., Gray, S., Lumsden, M. A., Marsden, J., Stevenson, J., et al. (2005). Managing the menopause: British Menopause Society Council consensus statement on hormone replacement therapy. *Journal of the British Menopause Society, 11,* 152–156.

Plomin, R., DeFries, J. C., McClearn, G. E., & Rutter, M. (2001). *Behavioral genetics* (4th ed.). New York: Freeman.

Pollack, M. H. (2005). Comorbid anxiety and depression. *Journal of Clinical Psychiatry, 66,* 22–29.

Pope, H. J., Jr. (1997). *Psychology astray: Fallacies in studies of "repressed memory" and childhood trauma.* Boca Raton, FL: Upton Books.

Prathikanti, S., & Weinberger, D. R. (2005). Psychiatric genetics—the new era: Genetic research and some clinical implications. *British Medical Bulletin, 73–74,* 107–122.

Prince, M. (1906). *The dissociation of a personality.* New York: Longmans, Green.

Ranz, J. M., Vergare, M. J., Wilk, J. E., Ackerman, S. H., Lippincott, R. C., Menninger, W. W., et al. (2006). The tipping point from private practice to publicly funded settings for early- and mid-career psychiatrists. *Psychiatric Services, 57,* 1640–1643.

Raymond, C. B., Morgan, S. G., & Caetano, P. A. (2007). Antidepressant utilization in British Columbia from 1996 to 2004: Increasing prevalence but not incidence. *Psychiatric Services, 58,* 79–84.

Razali, S. M. (2000). Masked depression: An ambiguous diagnosis. *Australian and New Zealand Journal of Psychiatry, 34,* 167.

Regestein, Q. R. (2000). Psychiatrists' views of managed care and the future of psychiatry. *General Hospital Psychiatry, 22,* 97–106.

Regier, D. A., Wilk, J., West, J. C., & Duffy, F. F. (2003, May). Current status of the psychiatry workforce in the United States. Presented at the American Psychiatric Association, San Francisco.

Reiber, R. W. (2006). *The bifurcation of the self.* New York: Springer.

Reik, T. (1951). *Listening with the third ear: The inner experience of a psycho-analyst.* Garden City, NY: Garden City Books.

Robins, E., & Guze, S. B. (1970). Establishment of diagnostic validity in psychiatric illness: Its application to schizophrenia. *American Journal of Psychiatry, 126,* 107–111.

Robins, L. N., & Regier, D. A. (Eds). (1991). *Psychiatric disorders in America.* New York: Free Press.

Robinson, D. (1996). *Wild beasts and idle humors: The insanity defense from antiquity to the present.* Cambridge: Harvard University Press.

Roseboom, P. H., & Kalin, N. H. (2000). Neuropharmacology of venlafaxine. *Depression & Anxiety, 12*(Suppl. 1), 20–29.

Rosenheck, R. (2005). The growth of psychopharmacology in the 1990's: Evidence-based practice or irrational exuberance? *International Journal of Law and Psychiatry, 28,* 467–483.

Rosenhecker, J., Huth, S., & Rudolph, C. (2006). Gene therapy for cystic fibrosis lung disease: Current status and future perspectives. *Current Opinion in Molecular Therapeutics, 8,* 439–445.

Rosenthal, D. (1971). *Genetics of psychopathology.* New York: McGraw Hill.

Rowland, A. S., Lesesne, C. A., & Abramowitz, A. J. (2002). The epidemiology of attention-deficit/hyperactivity disorder (ADHD): A public health view. *Mental Retardation & Developmental Disabilities Research Reviews, 8,* 162–170.

Rubinow, D. R. (2006). Treatment Strategies after SSRI Failure—Good News and Bad News. *New England Journal of Medicine, 354,* 1305–1307.

Rutter, M. (1987). Psychosocial resilience and protective mechanisms. *American Journal of Orthopsychiatry, 57,* 316–331.

Rutter, M., Kim-Cohen, J., & Maughan, B. (2006). Continuities and discontinuities in psychopathology between childhood and adult life. *Journal of Child Psychology & Psychiatry & Allied Disciplines, 47,* 276–295.

Rutter, M., Moffit, T. E., & Caspi, A. (2006). Gene-environment interplay and psychopathology: Multiple varieties but real effects. *Journal of Child Psychology & Psychiatry & Allied Disciplines, 47,* 226–261.

Rutter, M., & Rutter, M. (1993). *Developing minds: Challenge and continuity across the life span.* New York: Basic.

Rutter, M., & Smith, D. J. (1995). *Psychosocial disorders in young people: Time trends and their causes.* New York: Wiley.

Sackett, D. L., Rosenberg, W. M., Gray, J. A., Haynes, R. B., & Richardson, W. S. (1996). Evidence based medicine: What it is and what it isn't [editorial]. *British Medical Journal, 312*(7023), 71–72.

Sadler, J. Z. (2004). *Values and psychiatric diagnosis.* New York: Oxford University Press.

Sadock, B. J., Kaplan, H. I., & Sadock, V. A. (2004). *Kaplan and Sadock's comprehensive textbook of psychiatry* (8th ed.). Baltimore: Lippincott, Williams and Wilkins.

Salzman, C. (2005). The limited role of expert guidelines in teaching psychopharmacology. *Academic Psychiatry, 29,* 176–179.

Sandell, R., Blomberg, J., Lazar, A., Carlsson, J., Broberg, J., & Schubert, J. (2001). Varieties of long-term outcome among patients in psychoanalysis and long-term psychotherapy: A review of findings in the Stockholm Outcome of Psychoanalysis and Psychotherapy Project (STOPPP). *International Journal of Psychoanalysis, 82,* 205–210.

Sareen, J., Cox, B. J., Afifi, T. O., Yu, B. N., & Stein, M. B. (2005). Mental health service use in a nationally representative Canadian survey. *Canadian Journal of Psychiatry, 50,* 753–761.

Scarr, S., & McCartney, K. (1983). How people make their own environments: A theory of genotype-environment effects. *Child Development, 54,* 424–435.

Schacter, D. L. (1996). *Searching for memory.* New York: Basic.

Schatzberg, A., & Nemeroff, C. (2004). *The American Psychiatric Publishing textbook of psychopharmacology* (3rd ed.). Washington, DC: American Psychiatric Press.

Scheff, T. J. (1966). *Being mentally ill.* New York: Aldine.

Schimmel, P. (2001a). Mind over matter? I: Philosophical aspects of the mind-brain problem. *Australian & New Zealand Journal of Psychiatry, 35,* 481–487.

Schimmel, P. (2001b). Mind over matter? II: Implications for psychiatry. *Australian & New Zealand Journal of Psychiatry, 35,* 488–494.

Schoevers, R. A., Filip, D., Dorly, J. H., Cuijpers, P., Dekker, J., van Tilburg, W., Aartjan, T. F. (2006). Prevention of late-life depression in primary care: Do we know where to begin? *American Journal of Psychiatry, 163,* 1611–1621.

Schou, M. (2001). Lithium treatment at 52. *Journal of Affective Disorders, 67,* 21–32.

Schreiber, F. R. (1973). *Sybil.* Chicago: Regnery.

Schultz, W. (2006). Behavioral theories and the neurophysiology of reward. *Annual Review of Psychology, 57,* 87–115.

Scott, J., Paykel, E., Morriss, R., Bentall, R., Kinderman, P., & Johnson, T. (2006). Cognitive–behavioural therapy for severe and recurrent bipolar disorders. Randomised controlled trial. *British Journal of Psychiatry, 188,* 313–320.

Scully, J. H., & Wilk, J. E. (2003). Selected characteristics and data of psychiatrists in the United States, 2001–2002. *Academic Psychiatry, 27,* 247–251.

Searle, J. (2004). *Mind: A brief introduction.* Oxford, UK: Oxford University Press.

Seligman, M. E. P. (1995). The effectiveness of psychotherapy: The *Consumer Reports* study. *American Psychologist, 50,* 965–974.

Shea, M. T., Elkin, I., Imber, S. D., Sotsky, S. M., Watkins, J. T., Collins, J. F., Docherty, J. P. (1992). Course of depressive symptoms over follow-up: Findings from the National Institute of Mental Health Treatment of Depression Collaborative Research Program. *Archives of General Psychiatry, 49,* 782–787.

Shea, M. T., Pilkonis, P. A., Beckham, E., Collins, J. F., Elkin, E., Sotsky, S. M., et al. (1990). Personality disorders and treatment outcome in the NIMH Treatment of Depression Collaborative Research Program. *American Journal of Psychiatry, 147,* 711–718.

Shelton, C. I. (2004). Long-term management of major depressive disorder: Are differences among antidepressant treatments meaningful? *Journal of Clinical Psychiatry, 65*(Suppl. 17), 29–33.

Shorter, E. (1997). *A history of psychiatry.* New York: John Wiley.

Sierles, F. S., Dinwiddie, S. H., Patroi, D., Atre-Vaidya, N., Schrift, M. J., & Woodard, J. L. (2003). Factors affecting medical student career choice of psychiatry from 1999 to 2001. *Academic Psychiatry, 27,* 260–268.

Sierles, F. S., & Taylor, M. A. (1995). Decline of U.S. medical student career choice of psychiatry and what to do about it. *American Journal of Psychiatry, 152,* 1416–1426.

Siever, L. J., & Davis, K. L. (2004). The pathophysiology of schizophrenia disorders: Perspectives from the spectrum. *American Journal of Psychiatry, 161,* 398–413.

Siever, L. J., & Davis, K. L. (1991). A psychobiological perspective on the personality disorders. *American Journal of Psychiatry, 148,* 1647–1658.

Simon, R. I., & Gold, L. H. (Eds.). (2004). *The American Psychiatric Publishing textbook of forensic psychiatry.* Washington, DC: American Psychiatric Publishing.

Smith, M. L., Glass, G. V., & Miller, T. (1980). *The benefits of psychotherapy.* Baltimore: Johns Hopkins Press.

Spiegel, A. (2006, February 14). More and more, favored psychotherapy lets bygones be bygones. Retrieved December 20, 2006, from the *New York Times* Web site: http://nytimes.com.

Stein, D. J. (Ed.). (1997). *Cognitive science and the unconscious.* Washington, DC: American Psychiatric Press.

Stevens, J. C., & Pollack, M. H. (2005). Benzodiazepines in clinical practice: Consideration of their long-term use and alternative agents. *Journal of Clinical Psychiatry, 66*(Suppl. 2), 21–27.

Strupp, H. H. (1993). The Vanderbilt psychotherapy studies: Synopsis. *Journal of Consulting and Clinical Psychology, 61,* 431–433.

Strupp, H. H., Fox, R. E., & Lesser, K. (1969). *Patients view their psychotherapy.* Baltimore: Johns Hopkins Press.

Suarez, A. P., Marcus, S. C., Tanielian, T. L., & Pincus, H. A. (2001). Datapoints: Trends in psychiatric practice, 1988–1998: II. Caseload and treatment characteristics. *Psychiatric Services, 52,* 880.

Szasz, T. (1974). *The myth of mental illness* (Rev. ed.). New York: Harper and Row.

Szatmari, P. (2004). *A mind apart: Understanding children with autism and Asperger's syndrome.* New York: Guilford Press.

Szmukler, G., Dare, C., & Treasure, J. (Eds.). (1995). *Handbook of eating disorders: Theory, treatment and research.* Chichester, UK: John Wiley.

Tanielian, T. L., Marcus, S. C., Suarez, A. P., & Pincus, H. A. (2001). Datapoints: Trends in psychiatric practice, 1988–1998: III. Activities and work settings. *Psychiatric Services, 52,* 1026.

Tarrier, N. (2005). Cognitive behaviour therapy for schizophrenia: A review of development, evidence and implementation. *Psychotherapy & Psychosomatics, 74,* 136–144.

Taylor, M. J., & Goodwin, G. M. (2006). Long-term prophylaxis in bipolar disorder. *CNS Drugs, 20,* 303–310.

Thapar, A., O'Donovan, M., & Owen, M. J. (2005). The genetics of attention deficit hyperactivity disorder. *Human Molecular Genetics, 14*(Review Issue 2), R275–R282.

Thase, M. E. (2004). Therapeutic alternatives for difficult-to-treat depression: A narrative review of the state of the evidence. *CNS Spectrums, 9,* 808–816, 818–821.

Thase, M. E., Friedman, E. S., Biggs, M. M., Wisniewski, S. R., Trivedi, M. H., Luther, J. F., Fava, M., Nierenberg, A. A., McGrath, P. J., Warden, D., Niederehe, G., Hollon, S. D., & Rush, A. J. (2007). Cognitive therapy versus medication in augmentation and switch strategies as second-step treatments: A STAR*D report. *American Journal of Psychiatry, 164,* 739–752.

Thigpen, C. H., & Cleckley, H. M. (1957). *The three faces of Eve.* New York: McGraw-Hill.

Torrens, M., Fonseca, F., Mateu, G., & Farre, M. (2005). Efficacy of antidepressants in substance use disorders with and without comorbid depression. A systematic review and meta-analysis. *Drug & Alcohol Dependence, 78,* 1–22.

Torrey, E. F. (1988). *Nowhere to Go: The tragic odyssey of the homeless mentally ill.* New York: Harper and Row.

Trivedi, M. H., DeBattista, C., Fawcett, J., Nelson, C., Osser, D. N., Stein, D., et al. (1998). Developing treatment algorithms for unipolar depression in Cyberspace: International Psychopharmacology Algorithm Project (IPAP). *Psychopharmacology Bulletin, 34*(3), 355–359.

Trivedi, M. H., Fava, M., Wisniewski, S. R., Thase, M. E., Quitkin, F., Warden, D., et al. (2006). Medication augmentation after the failure of SSRIs for depression. *New England Journal of Medicine, 354,* 1243–1252.

True, W. R., Rice, J., Eisen, S. A., Heath, A. C., Goldberg, J., & Lyons, M. J. (1993). A twin study of genetic and environmental contributions to liability for post traumatic stress symptoms. *Archives of General Psychiatry, 50,* 257–264.

Turkington, D., Kingdon, D., & Weiden, P. J. (2006). Cognitive behavior therapy for schizophrenia. *American Journal of Psychiatry, 163,* 365–373.

Twyman, R. M. (2004). *Principles of proteomics.* New York: BIOS Scientific Publishers.

Valenstein, E. (1998). *Blaming the brain: The truth about drugs and mental illness.* New York: The Free Press.

van den Bree, M. B., & Owen, M. J. (2003). The future of psychiatric genetics. *Annals of Medicine, 35,* 122–134.

van Nimwegen, L., de Haan, L., van Beveren, N., van den Brink, W., & Linszen, D. (2005). Adolescence, schizophrenia and drug abuse: A window of vulnerability. *Acta Psychiatrica Scandinavica, Supplementum, 427,* 35–42.

Varan, L., Noiseux, R., Fleisher, W., Tomita, T., & Leverette, J. (2001). Medical training in psychiatric residency: The PGY–1 experience. *Canadian Journal of Psychiatry, 46,* 23.

Volkow, N. D., Wang, G. J., Fowler, J. S., & Ding, Y. S. (2005). Imaging the effects of methylphenidate on brain dopamine: New model on its therapeutic actions for attention-deficit/hyperactivity disorder. *Biological Psychiatry, 57,* 1410–1415.

von Bertalanffy, L. (1968). *General system theory: Foundations, developments, applications.* New York: Braziller.

Wakefield, J. C. (1992). Disorder as harmful dysfunction: A conceptual critique of DSM-III-R's definition of mental disorder. *Psychological Review, 99,* 232–247.

Wakefield, J. C., & First, M. (2003). Clarifying the distinction between disorder and non-disorder: Confronting the overdiagnosis ("false positives") problem in DSM-V. In K. A. Phillips, M. B. First, & H. A. Pincus (Eds.), *Advancing DSM: Dilemmas in psychiatric diagnosis* (pp. 23–56). Washington, DC: American Psychiatric Press.

Wakefield, J. C., Horwitz, A. V., & Schmitz, M. F. (2005). Are we over-pathologizing the socially anxious? Social phobia from a harmful dysfunction perspective. *Canadian Journal of Psychiatry, 50,* 317–319.

Wakefield, J. C., Schmitz, M. F., First, M. B., & Horwitz, A. (2007): Extending the bereavement exclusion for major depression to other losses. *Archives of General Psychiatry, 64,* 43–440.

Walsh, B. T., & Klein, D. A. (2003). Eating disorders. *International Review of Psychiatry, 15,* 205–216.

Walsh, J. (1923). *Cures: The story of the cures that fail.* New York: D. Appleton.

Wampold, B. E. (2001). *The great psychotherapy debate: Models, methods, and findings.* Mahwah, NJ: Erlbaum Associates.

Waraich, P., Goldner, E. M., Somers, J. M., & Hsu, L. (2004). Prevalence and incidence studies of mood disorders: A systematic review of the literature. *Canadian Journal of Psychiatry, 49,* 124–138.

Weiss, G., & Hechtman, L. (1993). *Hyperactive children grown up, second edition: ADHD in children, adolescents, and adults.* New York: Guilford Press.

Weissman, M. M., & Klerman, G. L. (1993). *New applications of interpersonal therapy.* Washington, DC: American Psychiatric Press.

Weissman, M. M., Verdeli, H., Gameroff, M. J., Bledsoe, S. E., Betts, K., Mufson, L., et al. (2006). National survey of psychotherapy training in psychiatry, psychology, and social work. *Archives of General Psychiatry, 63*, 925–934.

Weissman, S. (1996). Recruitment and workforce issues in late 20th century American psychiatry. *Psychiatric Quarterly, 67*, 125–137.

Wender, P. (2000). *ADHD: Attention-deficit hyperactivity disorder in children, adolescents, and adults.* Oxford: Oxford University Press.

Westen, D. (2006). Are research patients and clinical trials representative of clinical practice? In J. C. Norcross, L. E. Beutler, & R. F. Levant (Eds.). *Evidence-based practices in mental health: Debate and dialogue on the fundamental questions* (pp. 161–189). Washington, DC: American Psychological Association.

Westen, D. (1999). The scientific status of unconscious processes: Is Freud really dead? *Journal of the American Psychoanalytical Association, 47*, 1061–1106.

Wilk, J. E., West, J. C., Narrow, W. E., Rae, D. S., & Regier, D. A. (2005). Economic grand rounds: Access to psychiatrists in the public sector and in managed health plans. *Psychiatric Services, 56*, 408–410.

Wilk, J. E., West, J. C., Rae, D. S., & Regier, D. A. (2006). Patterns of adult psychotherapy in psychiatric practice. *Psychiatric Services, 57*, 472–476.

Yager, J. (2002). The 2002 psychologist prescribing law in New Mexico: The psychiatrists' perspective. *Maryland Medicine, 3*, 21–23.

Yehuda, R. (1999). Biological factors associated with susceptibility to posttraumatic stress disorder. *Canadian Journal of Psychiatry, 44*, 34–39.

Yehuda, R., & McFarlane, A. C. (1995). Conflict between current knowledge about posttraumatic stress disorder and its original conceptual basis. *American Journal of Psychiatry, 152*, 1705–1713.

Young, A. (1995). *The harmony of illusions: Inventing posttraumatic stress disorder.* Princeton, NJ: Princeton University Press.

Zanarini, M. C. (1993). Borderline personality as an impulse spectrum disorder. In J. Paris (Ed.), *Borderline personality disorder: Etiology and treatment* (pp. 67–86). Washington, DC: American Psychiatric Press.

Zanarini, M. C., Frankenburg, F. R., Khera, G. S., & Bleichmar, J. (2001). Treatment histories of borderline inpatients. *Comprehensive Psychiatry, 42*, 144–150.

Zimmerman, M., Rothschild, L., & Chelminski, I. (2005). The prevalence of DSM-IV personality disorders in psychiatric outpatients. *American Journal of Psychiatry, 162*(10), 1911–1918.

Index